DRUG RESISTANCE

SWOSU-Sayre / McMahan Library

Recent Titles in
Health and Medical Issues Today

Medicare
Jennie Jacobs Kronenfeld

Illicit Drugs
Richard E. Isralowitz and Peter L. Myers

Animal-Assisted Therapy
Donald Altschiller

Alcohol
Peter L. Myers and Richard E. Isralowitz

Geriatrics
Carol Leth Stone

Plastic Surgery
Lana Thompson

Birth Control
Aharon W. Zorea

Bullying
Sally Kuykendall, PhD

Steroids
Aharon W. Zorea

Suicide and Mental Health
Rudy Nydegger

Cutting and Self-Harm
Chris Simpson

Discrimination Against the Mentally Ill
Monica A. Joseph

Concussions
William Paul Meehan III

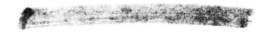

DRUG RESISTANCE

Sarah E. Boslaugh

Health and Medical Issues Today

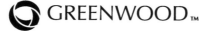 GREENWOOD™

An Imprint of ABC-CLIO, LLC
Santa Barbara, California • Denver, Colorado

Copyright © 2017 by ABC-CLIO, LLC

All rights reserved. No part of this publication may be reproduced, stored in a retrieval system, or transmitted, in any form or by any means, electronic, mechanical, photocopying, recording, or otherwise, except for the inclusion of brief quotations in a review, without prior permission in writing from the publisher.

Library of Congress Cataloging-in-Publication Data

Names: Boslaugh, Sarah.
Title: Drug resistance / Sarah E. Boslaugh.
Description: Santa Barbara, California : Greenwood, an imprint of ABC-CLIO, LLC,
  [2017] | Series: Health and medical issues today | Includes bibliographical references
  and index.
Identifiers: LCCN 2016038910 (print) | LCCN 2016041055 (ebook) |
  ISBN 9781440839245 (hard copy : alk. paper) | ISBN 9781440839252 (ebook)
Subjects: LCSH: Drug resistance. | Antibiotics.
Classification: LCC QR177 .B67 2017 (print) | LCC QR177 (ebook) |
  DDC 616.9/041—dc23
LC record available at https://lccn.loc.gov/2016038910

ISBN: 978-1-4408-3924-5
EISBN: 978-1-4408-3925-2

21 20 19 18   3 4 5

This book is also available as an eBook.

Greenwood
An Imprint of ABC-CLIO, LLC

ABC-CLIO, LLC
130 Cremona Dr., P.O. Box 1911
Santa Barbara, CA 93116-1911
www.abc-clio.com

This book is printed on acid-free paper ∞

Manufactured in the United States of America

This book is dedicated to my colleagues, students, and professors, because science is truly a collaborative endeavor.

CONTENTS

Series Foreword   xi

Acknowledgments   xiii

Introduction   xv

**Section I: Overview and Historical Background
              of Drug Resistance**   **1**

 1   The Science of Drug Resistance   3
       What Are Antimicrobials?   3
       Key Antibiotics in Medical History   7
       What Is Antimicrobial Resistance?   13
       How Microbes Become Resistant   14
       Why Drug Resistance Is a Concern   16

 2   The Role of Human Behavior in Drug Resistance   19
       Inappropriate Use of Drugs   19
       Use of Low-Quality Drugs   23
       Use of Antimicrobials in Animal Husbandry   24

 3   The Scope of the Problem Today   25
       Global Overview of Drug Resistance   25
       Drug Resistance in the United States   34

 4   Specific Diseases   43
       Tuberculosis   43
       Gonorrhea   46

	Malaria	48
	HIV	51
	Influenza	53

5	Measures to Combat Drug Resistance	57
	National and International Standards of Prescribing Practice	57
	Infection Control	65
	Vaccination Programs	68
	Limiting Disease Spread through Travel	69
	Developing New Antibiotics and Improved Diagnostic Tests	72
	Surveillance and Reporting Programs	73
	Recommendations for Global Surveillance	75

| **Section II: Contemporary Issues and Debates** | | **77** |

6	Drug Resistance as a National and International Issue	79
	Stakeholders	80
	Recommendations for Antibiotic Use	81
	Developing New Antibiotics	87

7	Changing Physician and Pharmacist Behavior	95
	Decision Making in Medicine	96
	Physician and Pharmacist Education	97
	Health System Guidelines	100

8	Changing Patient Behavior	103
	Patient Adherence	103
	Obstacles to Adherence	106
	Interventions to Improve Adherence	108

9	Balancing Individual and Societal Rights	111
	Balancing Infection Control and the Right to Freedom and Privacy	111
	DOT	112
	Involuntary Quarantine	114

10	Contributions of Research to the Fight Against Drug Resistance	121
	The Drug Development Process	121
	Antibiotics in the Drug Development Pipeline	125

11	Antibiotics in Animal Husbandry	127
	History	129
	Specific Threats	130

The Scope of the Issue   132
Balancing Productivity and Public Safety   135

Section III: Resources   **139**

Primary Documents   141
  Current Reports   141
    Antimicrobial Resistance: Global Report
    on Surveillance: Summary   141
    Antibiotic Resistance Threats in the United States, 2013:
    Executive Summary   147
    Antimicrobial Resistance Surveillance in Europe, 2015:
    Summary   149
  Policy Statements   153
    WHO Global Strategy for Containment of Antimicrobial
    Resistance: Executive Summary   153
    National Strategy for Combating Antibiotic Resistance
    Bacteria: Executive Summary   161
    The Judicious Use of Medically Important
    Antimicrobial Drugs in Food-Producing Animals:
    Executive Summary   166

Timeline   175

Sources for Further Information   185

Glossary   197
Index   203

SERIES FOREWORD

Every day, the public is bombarded with information on developments in medicine and healthcare. Whether it is about the latest techniques in treatment or research, or concerns over public health threats, this information directly affects the lives of people more than almost any other issue. Although there are many sources for understanding these topics—from Web sites and blogs to newspapers and magazines—people often need one resource that makes sense of the complex health and medical issues affecting their daily lives.

The *Health and Medical Issues Today* series provides just such a one-stop resource for obtaining a solid overview of the most controversial areas of healthcare in the 21st century. Each volume addresses one topic and provides a balanced summary of what is known. These volumes provide an excellent first step for students and laypeople interested in understanding how healthcare works in our society today.

Each volume is broken into several sections to provide readers and researchers with easy access to the information they need:

- Section I provides overview chapters on background information, including chapters on such areas as the historical, scientific, medical, social, and legal issues involved—that a citizen needs to intelligently understand the topic.
- Section II provides capsule examinations of the most heated contemporary issues and debates and analyzes in a balanced manner the viewpoints held by various advocates in the debates.

- Section III provides a selection of reference materials, such as annotated primary source documents, a timeline of important events, and a directory of organizations that serve as the best next step in learning about the topic at hand.

The *Health and Medical Issues Today* series strives to provide readers with all the information needed to begin making sense of some of the most important debates going on in the world today. The series includes volumes on such topics as stem-cell research, obesity, gene therapy, alternative medicine, organ transplantation, mental health, and more.

ACKNOWLEDGMENTS

Much of the information incorporated in this book comes from data collected and reported by governmental organizations such as the Centers for Disease Control and Prevention (CDC), and from the World Health Organization (WHO), an agency of the United Nations. Without their tireless work, our ability to understand key medical and health issues would be far less than it is today.

INTRODUCTION

Modern medicine is able to cure or contain many diseases that posed a serious threat to human life less than a century ago. Many of these great breakthroughs were made possible by the development of new drugs, including
antibiotics such as penicillin and streptomycin, that were rightly hailed as
miracle drugs when first introduced into medical use. Other drugs have been
developed that are effective against diseases caused by means other than
bacteria, such as malaria, which is caused by infection with a parasite, and
acquired immune deficiency syndrome (AIDS), which is caused by a
viral infection.

However, these gains can be lost when disease-causing microorganisms
(e.g., bacteria and viruses) become resistant to drugs that formerly had been
effective against them. Often, a microorganism that develops resistance to
one drug remains susceptible to one or more other drugs, but as more and
more microorganisms become resistant to more and more drugs, the possibility increases for the emergence of microorganisms against which medical science has no effective remedy. This possibility is furthered by the
fact that the rate of discovery of new antibiotics today is much slower than
in the 1940s and 1950s, a period sometimes referred to as the *golden age
of antibiotics discovery*. Finally, even if alternatives exist to treat drug-
resistant organisms, these drugs are often more expensive and less readily
available, and they also may have more serious side effects than the drugs
that had been effective against the same organisms.

According to the World Health Organization (WHO), high rates of resistance to drugs ordinarily used to treat diseases caused by common types of
bacteria have been observed in all WHO regions. Among disease-causing

agents that have developed resistance to drugs formerly effective against them, those of greatest concern include *Escherichia coli*, which can cause serious infections in the bloodstream and urinary tract; *Klebsiella pneumoniae*, which can cause pneumonia, meningitis, and infections in wounds, the bloodstream, and the urinary tract; *Staphylococcus aureus*, which can cause infections of the skin, respiratory tract, bloodstream, and urinary tract; *Streptococcus pneumoniae*, which can cause pneumonia, meningitis, and otitis media (inner ear inflammation); *Salmonella*, which can cause food poisoning; *Shigella*, which can cause severe diarrhea and dysentery; and *Neisseria gonorrhoeae*, which causes the sexually transmitted disease gonorrhea.

Specific diseases for which drug resistance is of particular concern include tuberculosis (TB), which kills about 1.5 million people globally each year; malaria, which kills over 600,000 people annually, with an estimated 207 million seeking treatment each year; AIDS, which kills about 1.5 million people each year; and influenza, which kills 250,000 to 500,000 people annually. The death toll of these diseases would be even higher, of course, if the microorganisms causing them became resistant to the drugs available to treat them.

In part, the development of drug resistance is a natural process driven by selection pressure, but it may also be fostered by the way that antibiotics and other drugs are used. The emergence of drug-resistant strains of disease-causing microorganisms is often observed almost as soon as the drugs are used. For instance, streptomycin was introduced to medical care in 1946 as the first antibiotic effective against in treating TB patients; the same year, streptomycin-resistant strains of TB were found.

While drug resistance is a serious and growing threat to health, many things can be done to help limit or contain the growth of drug-resistant organisms and the human toll of disease caused by them. The means available to combat drug resistance include ending the overuse of antibiotics in human medicine; improving patient and provider education so that antibiotics are taken correctly; improving infection control procedures, particularly in hospitals and other health care settings; increasing vaccination programs; limiting the spread of disease through travel; developing new drugs; limiting or prohibiting the use of antibiotics as growth promoters in animal husbandry; and improving surveillance and reporting programs. None of these measures is cost free or easy to implement, and they require coordination and cooperation among many different stakeholders. However, drug resistance poses so serious a threat to human life that it is imperative that the stakeholders involved find ways to cooperate and develop effective measures to slow the growth of drug resistance and the spread of disease caused by resistant organisms.

Overview and Historical Background of Drug Resistance

CHAPTER 1

The Science of Drug Resistance

When a microorganism becomes *drug resistant*, that means that one or more drugs formerly effective in killing or inhibiting the growth of the microorganism are no longer effective against it. In medicine, this term means that one or more drugs formerly useful in treating or curing a disease caused by a particular microorganism no longer work effectively against that disease. To understand how an organism can become drug resistant, it is necessary to understand some basic facts about antimicrobials (of which antibiotic drugs are a specific type) and how they interact with microbes.

WHAT ARE ANTIMICROBIALS?

The term *antimicrobial* refers to chemicals or other substances or products that kill microorganisms or slow their rate of growth. Antimicrobials are classified according to the type of microorganism that they are effective against. Types of antimicrobials include antibacterials, which are used against bacteria; antivirals, which are used against viruses; antifungals, which are used against funguses; antimycobacterials, which are used against mycobacteria; and antiparasitics, which are used against parasites. Note that the terms *antibacterial* and *antibiotic* are sometimes treated as synonyms, and the antibiotic type of antimicrobial is most familiar to many people because of the many antibiotics, such as penicillin and tetracycline, used in medicine.

Many different antimicrobials are used today, with some being effective against a broad class of microorganisms (broad-spectrum antimicrobials), and others being effective against a smaller subset of microorganisms (narrow-spectrum antimicrobials). Antimicrobials used in medicine may have multiple names, including a generic name (e.g., cephalexin) and one or more brand names (e.g., Keflex, Panixine, Biocef, Zartan). Different antimicrobials within a particular type are often grouped into classes based on chemical similarity, so that ofloxacin and levofloxacin both belong to the fluoroquinolone class, while amoxicillin and ampicillin both belong to the penicillin class.

There are many ways that antimicrobials can attack and kill or contain the growth of microbes. Looking just at antibiotics, penicillin kills bacteria by damaging and penetrating the cell walls of bacteria, while vancomycin inhibits the ability of bacteria to form cell walls. Fluoroquinolones affect the deoxyribonucleic acid (DNA) in the microbe's cells, causing it to fragment, while tetracyclines affect the ribonucleic acid (RNA) and inhibit protein synthesis. The key points are that antimicrobials have different effects on different microbes, and the development of antibiotic resistance involves the microbe developing in a way that prevents a particular effect or effects from occurring.

Although people often think of antimicrobials, and antibiotics in particular, as referring to pharmaceuticals (drugs) meant for human consumption, many other common products also have antimicrobial properties, and the same antimicrobial may be used for multiple purposes. For instance, bleach is a common name for products containing sodium hypochlorite (NaCIO), usually as a solution with water. Bleach is a broad-spectrum antimicrobial that is commonly used as a disinfectant in both homes and commercial and public places (e.g., hospitals, swimming pools, and restaurants). Besides its disinfectant properties, bleach has many other uses, from removing stains from laundry to treating wood pulp during the process of making paper.

The National Pesticide Information Center at Oregon State University divides antimicrobial products used in public health into three categories: Sanitizers, disinfectants, and sterilizers (listed in increasing order of strength). *Sanitizers* are used on surfaces (e.g., kitchen counters and toilets) to reduce the number of bacteria on the surface, with some intended for use only on surfaces that will *not* come into contact with food. *Disinfectants* are used to kill or prevent the growth of microbes and are commonly used in health care settings as well as home use, but they cannot be used on surfaces that will come into contact with food. Note that this distinction is not always observed in practice—sometimes products advertised as disinfectants are in fact intended for use on food preparation surfaces. Disinfectants can be subdivided further into *microbistats*, which slow the growth of microbes without killing them, and *microbicides*, which kill microbes. Sterilizers include some types of pesticides and kill spores (primitive reproductive bodies that can give rise to new organisms) as well as microbes. Sterilizers are frequently used in medical and research settings, where high priority is given to removing all traces of microbes.

Classes of Antibiotics

Within the category of antibiotics, there are many different classes of drugs. For instance, while it is common to speak of "penicillin" as if it were a single drug, there is in fact a category of drugs that are chemically similar and also are called "penicillin." One reason that it is necessary to have so many classes of antibiotics is that a wide variety of microbes can cause disease, and no single class of antibiotic is effective against all microbes or in treating all diseases. To cite one example, penicillins are effective in treating strep throat, but not tuberculosis (TB). Here are some of the major classes of antibiotics, listing some of the drugs in each class (note the similarities among names of specific drugs in each class—you often can deduce the class of antibiotic from the name of a specific drug):

- Penicillins: Amoxicillin, flucloxacillin, methicillin (also called *meticillin*)
- Cephalosporins: Cephalexin, cefaclor, cefotetan
- Carbapenems: Meropenem, imipenem, doripenem
- Tetracyclines: Tetracycline, doxycycline, minocycline
- Macrolides: Erythromycin, azithromycin, clarithromycin
- Quinolones: Ciprofloxacin, norfloxacin, levofloxacin

Different drugs within each class have been developed over the years. The earliest drugs in each class are sometimes referred to as "first-generation," as in "first-generation cephalosporins," with later drugs within the class referred to as "second-generation," "third-generation," and so on. When a microbe becomes resistant to a first-generation drug, it is possible that it will be susceptible to the second-generation version of the same drug because there may be enough differences between the drugs from different generations that resistance to the first does not equate to resistance to the second. For this reason, drug resistance is often specified with regard to the generation as well as the type of the drug. For instance, the World Health Organization (WHO) reports that *Klebsiella pneumoniae*, a bacteria that can cause pneumonia, urinary tract infections, and other diseases, has developed resistance to third-generation cephalorosporins, with reports of at least 50 percent resistance coming from countries in all six WHO regions.

The progress of drug resistance, and the necessity of having a wide variety of treatment options (and developing new options), can be seen from the history of the drug class known as *β-lactams*, or *Beta-lactams*. This class of drugs includes the penicillins, cephalosporins, and carbapenems, which are commonly used to treat gram-negative infections. Although the penicillins were among the first antibiotics developed and were originally effective against a number of pathogens, they are less effective today because many microorganisms have developed resistance to them. The cephalosporins were developed more recently and have been a mainstay of the treatment of resistant gram-negative infections, but they are becoming less effective as resistance to their effects becomes more widespread. The third type of *β-lactam*, the carbapenems, is currently the treatment of last resort for infections caused by gram-negative bacteria resistant to both penicillins and cephalosporins. However, infection with bacteria resistant to carbapenems has been identified in both the United States and other countries, and given the natural tendency of bacteria to develop resistance, infections with carbapenem-resistant bacteria can be expected to increase in the future. Once a pathogen becomes resistant to carbapenems, it is generally resistant to all drugs in the *β-lactam* class, meaning that no drug in this category can be used to treat infections caused by that pathogen.

Gram-Positive and Gram-Negative Bacteria

One broad method of classifying bacteria is as gram-positive or gram-negative. These classifications reflect the way that various types of bacteria respond to a laboratory method called *Gram staining*, a procedure developed by the Danish bacteriologist Hans Christian Gram in the late 19th century). In Gram staining, microorganisms are exposed to two dyes called crystal violet and safranin. The way that the organisms respond to those dyes results in their classification as gram positive (which are stained purple as a result of the process) or gram negative (which are stained pink). Gram staining is often the first step to test for the presence of bacteria in an infection, and to identify the type of bacteria if it is present, in order to plan medical treatment for the infection.

Gram-positive and gram-negative bacteria differ in ways that affect how they respond to various antibiotics. The cell walls of gram-positive bacteria include a thick layer of peptidoglycan (a complex combination of sugars and proteins), while gram-positive bacteria have a much thinner layer of peptidoglycan in their cell walls. Gram-negative cells also have an outer layer or membrane made of proteins, lipids, and polysaccharides, while gram-positive cells do not have this outer membrane. The presence of this outer membrane makes gram-negative bacteria less vulnerable to many types of antibiotics than gram-positive bacteria.

Examples of types of gram-positive bacteria include *streptococcus* (which can cause diseases such as strep throat, bacterial pneumonia, and rheumatic fever), *staphylococcus* (which can cause diseases such as food poisoning, toxic shock syndrome, and staphylococcal meningitis), *bacillus* (which can cause diseases such as anthrax and food poisoning), *corynebacteria* (which can cause diseases such as diphtheria and endocarditis) and *clostridium* (which can cause diseases such as botulism and tetanus). Examples of types of gram-negative bacteria include *pseudomonadaceae* (which can cause urinary tract infections and burn infections), and *enterobacteriaceae* (which can cause diseases such as plague, salmonellosis, and *Klebsiella* pneumonia).

In terms of antimicrobial resistance, the greatest threat is posed by gram-negative bacteria because some bacteria in this class have displayed resistance to nearly all the drugs available to treat them. Some of the most serious healthcare-acquired infections are caused by gram-negative pathogens, including various *Enterobacter*, *Pseudomonas*, and *Acinetobacter* species. *Acinetobacter* are commonly found on the skin, can be life-threatening for people with compromised immune systems, and are a common cause of pneumonia contracted by patients in intensive care units, particularly those using ventilators.

KEY ANTIBIOTICS IN MEDICAL HISTORY

Carbolic Acid

Carbolic acid, also known as *phenol*, is a compound of carbon, hydrogen, and oxygen with the chemical formula C_6H_5OH. A solution of carbolic acid in water has antimicrobial properties, and carbolic acid was the first topical antimicrobial to be incorporated into medical practice to reduce the rate of infection from surgery. In Europe in the mid-19th century, it was common for a patient to survive a surgical procedure, only to die of an infection after the surgery was completed. The British surgeon Joseph Lister believed that the cause of these infections were microorganisms that entered the body through incisions made during surgery. To combat these infections, he cleaned patients' wounds with carbolic acid and dressed them with bandages soaked in carbolic acid. He also required surgeons to wash their hands with carbolic acid, used carbolic acid to clean surgical tools, and developed a technique to spray a carbolic acid solution into the air of the operating theater.

The benefits of these antiseptic procedures were immediately evident: The death rate for Lister's surgical patients dropped from 45 percent in

1864–1866, before he began using carbolic acid during surgery, to 15 percent in 1867–1870, after he instituted the carbolic acid procedures. Today, carbolic acid is no longer used in surgical practice in the ways that he used it, in part because it is so harsh that it can damage skin tissues. However, Lister's work established the principle that using topical antiseptics could prevent infection during surgery. His work also paved the way for modern sterile practices in surgery, and more generally for the importance of effective antiseptic practices in hospitals.

Salversan

One of the first successful antibiotics, Salversan, was developed by the German physician Paul Ehrlich and introduced to medical practice in 1910. Ehrlich was searching for a treatment for syphilis, a sexually transmitted disease caused by the spirochete (spiral-shaped) bacterium *Treponema pallidum pallidum*. At the time, there was no effective treatment for syphilis, a dreaded disease that could result in consequences including sores and skin ulcers, severe pain, tumors, and dementia. Syphilis is now known to have existed in Europe since at least 1495, and it was feared in Western societies similar to how HIV/AIDS was feared before the introduction of effective antiretroviral therapies. Prior to the introduction of Salversan, patients were treated with mercury, but these treatments were not always effective and also often resulted in the patient becoming ill from mercury poisoning.

Ehrlich's research was focused on finding a specific drug to treat a specific condition. During his medical studies, he noted that certain dyes could be used to stain specific microbes, and he imagined that drugs could be developed in a similar way, so that they targeted a particular microbe. He referred to this quest to develop targeted treatments as the search for a "magic bullet" that would kill the microbes causing disease but not otherwise cause harm to the patient. Such a treatment would stand in sharp contrast to, for instance, the mercury treatments for syphilis then in use, which had many ill effects on patients, including loss of teeth, mouth ulcers, and kidney failure.

Ehrlich, working with a team of scientists including the German chemist Alfred Bertheim and the Japanese bacteriologist Sahachiro Hata, created and tested hundreds of organic arsenic compounds before arriving in 1909 at arsphenamine, which cured syphilis-infected rabbits with a single dose. Arsphenamine was also known in the lab as "Compound 606" (reflecting its place among the many compounds tested by the research team) and was brought to market in 1910 under the brand name Salversan. As the first effective treatment for syphilis, Salversan quickly became the most widely prescribed drug in the world and remained the standard treatment for syphilis until the introduction of penicillin in the 1940s.

Penicillin

The first broad-spectrum antibiotic, penicillin, was discovered in 1928 by the Scottish physician and researcher Alexander Fleming. Penicillin was also the first antibiotic discovered from a natural source, rather than being created in the lab. In contrast to Ehrlich's purposeful search for a drug that would be effective against a specific illness, Fleming's discovery of penicillin had its beginnings in a happy accident. Fleming was cleaning up his lab when he noticed an odd pattern on a glass plate. The plate had been coated with a *staphylococcus* (staph) bacteria culture, but it also had a bit of mold on it. Fleming noted that the area around the moldy spot was free of the staph culture, and he conducted further experiments to investigate the properties of the mold, which he later called *penicillium notatum* (today known as *penicillium chrysogenum*) or penicillin. He discovered that even an extremely dilute solution of penicillin could prevent the growth of staph. Although Fleming published an article about his discovery in 1919, it did not attract a great deal of scientific attention.

Penicillin is an interesting case study that highlights the steps beyond initial discovery that are required before a drug becomes useful in a clinical sense. To put it another way, an interesting discovery in the lab does not immediately translate to a new drug being commonly available to treat patients. The outbreak of World War II meant that there was great interest in producing penicillin to treat soldiers. However, Fleming did not have the lab resources or expertise to undertake the tasks necessary to isolate and purify the active ingredient, test its effectiveness against different microbes, and develop a way to produce it in large quantities. To hasten the process of making penicillin available to treat patients, Sir Howard Walter Florey, director of the School of Pathology at Oxford University, and Florey's protogé Ernest Boris Chain, a Jewish émigré from Germany, took up the work of creating a method to produce penicillin in clinically useful quantities. Their first test case, in 1940, involved treating a patient infected with both streptococci and staphylococci through a cut in his skin. The infection was resistant to the sulfa drugs then in use, but the patient began to recover after being treated with penicillin. However, the supply of penicillin ran out after five days, and the patient worsened and died.

The biochemist Norman Heatley, working in the same lab as Florey and Chain, also worked on ways to refine penicillin and produce it in large quantities. In 1941, Florey and Heatley came to the United States to work with

American scientists on the problem of mass-producing penicillin. Their efforts were successful, and American pharmaceutical companies produced 400 million units of pure penicillin in the first five months of 1942. By 1945, penicillin production had increased to 650 billion units per month, and the effectiveness of this "wonder drug" was proven by the substantial reduction in deaths due to infection among soldiers who were treated with penicillin. In 1945, Fleming, Florey, and Chain were awarded the Nobel Prize in Physiology or Medicine for their work with penicillin.

Besides his scientific accomplishments, Fleming was ahead of his time in predicting that the era of miracle cures made possible by penicillin might not last. In a 1945 interview with the *New York Times*, he warned that the ability of penicillin to fight infection could be compromised by misusing it. His prediction came true: within 10 years after the wide-scale introduction of penicillin to treat civilians, many types of bacteria had begun to develop resistance to it.

Sulfa Drugs

Sulfa drugs, also called *sulfonamides*, were introduced for medical use in 1935, making them the first widely available antibiotics for human use. Sulfa drugs are all related to the compound sulfanilamide, an organic compound consisting of a sulfonamide group and an aniline. Sulfanilimide was developed by the Austrian scientist Paul Gelmo as part of his dissertation research, and it was patented in 1935. However, the first antibacterial drug based on sulfanilamide, Prontosil, was developed by the German scientist Gerhard Domagk while working in the pharmaceuticals division of I.G. Farben, an industry conglomerate specializing in chemical compounds and dyes.

Domagk tested hundreds of compounds for their antibacterial properties. One such compound, KL 695, proved to be useful in treating lab mice infected with streptococcus. Working with two colleagues, Fritz Mietzsch and Josef Klarer, Domagk altered the chemical makeup of this compound and produced KL 730, which had much stronger antibacterial properties. They patented this compound under the name Prontosil, and Domagk published the results of his studies on this compound in 1935. By this time, Prontosil had already been used to treat both staph and strep infections in humans, including a case of strep infection in Domagyk's own daughter.

Domagk was awarded the Nobel Prize in Physiology or Medicine in 1939 for his work with Prontosil, and sulfa drugs were developed to treat many conditions, including burns, blood poisoning, meningitis, and pneumonia. The emergence of penicillin as a highly effective, broad-spectrum antibiotic meant that sulfa drugs became less important in treating infections, although they still remain in use today, alone or in combination with other drugs. For instance, sulfadiazine is commonly used to treat urinary tract infections, and the combination of erythromycin and sulfafurazole, which make up the branded drug Pediazole, is used to treat ear infections in children.

Streptomycin

Penicillin was rightly hailed as a wonder drug because it could effectively treat many infectious diseases that had previously been life-threatening. However, it was ineffective against one infectious disease that was widespread at the time: TB. TB is an ancient disease: some Egyptian mummies show evidence of tubercular infection, and the disease is mentioned in the books of Deuteronomy and Leviticus in the Bible. The Greek physician Hippocrates (c.460 BCE–370 BCE) described TB, and archaeological evidence suggests that it was also found in the Americas long before the arrival of Columbus. In the 19th century, both Europe and the United States experienced TB epidemics, and various methods to treat patients were developed, including sending patients to special TB hospitals (called *sanitoriums*), which were located in the mountains because the air was believed to be healthier in such regions.

Modern understanding of TB dates to 1882, when the German physician Hermann Heinrich Robert Koch presented and published research demonstrating that the causal agent of TB is *mycobacterium tuberculosis*, also referred to as the *tubercle bacillus*. Two therapeutic agents with some effectiveness against TB, para-aminosalicylic acid (PAS) and thiosemicarbazone, were discovered in the 1940s. However, these drugs were only bacteriostatic, meaning that they prevented the TB bacilli from reproducing but did not kill the existing bacilli. The great breakthrough in TB treatment came in 1944, when a research group led by the Ukrainian Jewish émigré Selman Abraham Waksman discovered streptomycin, the first antibiotic effective against TB. Waksman's group worked at Rutgers University, but his lab did not have the facilities to conduct the necessary tests to bring streptomycin to market, so testing was carried out at the Mayo Clinic in Rochester, Minnesota.

The effectiveness of streptomycin in treating TB was confirmed in both animal models and clinical trials. It also proved to be useful for treating a number of other diseases, including typhoid, cholera, tularemia, and urinary tract infections. Some of the research necessary to develop streptomycin was funded by the pharmaceutical manufacturer Merck in return for an exclusive license to produce the drug. However, when Waksman realized what an important drug streptomycin could be, in terms of fighting disease and reducing human suffering, he appealed to Merck to allow other pharmaceutical companies to produce streptomycin as well. His concern was twofold: he was afraid that Merck might not be able to meet the demand for this new drug, and he felt the price of the drug would be higher if only one company produced it. Merck agreed to accept a nonexclusive license to produce streptomycin, and several other pharmaceutical manufacturers also began producing the drug.

Numerous drugs are available to treat TB today, including isoniazid, discovered in 1952, and rifampin, discovered in 1967. Thanks to the availability of effective antibiotics, TB in the developed world (including high- and middle-income industrialized countries such as the United States and the United Kingdom) quickly went from being a dreaded scourge treated in special hospitals to a curable disease treated with ordinary medical care. As the number of people with active TB declined in populations, so did rates of infection, and TB became relatively rare. However, it remains a major health threat in developing countries (i.e., low-income countries with a low level of development), while the rise of drug-resistant TB means that the disease is once again a concern of health systems in the developed world as well.

Antibiotic Use Today

Antibiotics remain one of the most important weapons that modern medicine can use to fight human disease. A wide variety of antibiotics and other antimicrobial medicines (e.g., antiparasitics, used to combat diseases caused by parasites) are widely used throughout the world. The most recent edition of the WHO's *Model List of Essential Medicines*, which includes medicines that have been evaluated for their efficacy, safety, cost-effectiveness, and usefulness in combating health threats, includes many antibiotics. Many countries use the *Model List* as a guide to deciding what medicines should be granted the highest priority in terms of making them available to their citizens.

There is no single source of information on antibiotic use worldwide, and even within a single country, it may be difficult to determine the level of antibiotic use for a given year. However, surveys and analyses of administrative data (e.g., records of pharmaceutical sales) can provide estimates of antibiotic sales (which can be used to provide estimates of antibiotic use) and also provide a way to track changes in estimated antibiotic sales and use. Thomas P. Van Boeckel and colleagues analyzed sales data from retail and hospital pharmacies in 63 countries and found several patterns of interest. First, consumption of antibiotic drugs increased 36 percent between 2000 and 2010, with 76 percent of the increase seen in only five countries:

Brazil, Russia, India, China, and South Africa, the so-called BRICS countries (because of the first letters of their names), all of which have large populations and fast-growing economies. With the exception of Australia and New Zealand, antibiotic use was fairly steady or declined in most developed countries during this period.

In both 2000 and 2010, the antibiotics most commonly used were broad-spectrum antibiotics, followed by cephalosporins, macrolides, fluoroquinolones, trimethoprim, tetracyclines, and narrow-spectrum penicillins, with broad-spectrum penicillins and cephalosporins alone accounting for over half (55 percent) of antibiotic use in 2010. India was the largest consumer of antibiotics in 2010, followed by China and the United States. Per capita (per person) use of antibiotics varied widely even among countries with similar levels of economic development: for instance, in 2010, France used about three times as many antibiotics per capita as did the Netherlands. Many countries showed strong seasonal patterns in antibiotic use, with use peaking in the colder months (January through March in the northern hemisphere, July through September in the southern hemisphere) or, in the case of India, at the end of the monsoon season (July and September).

A study of antibiotic use in European countries in 2012, conducted by the European Centre for Disease Convention and Control (ECDC), found that antibiotics were commonly used in most countries surveyed, but that there were also wide variations in the amount of antibiotics used from one country to another. This survey, which includes most western and northern European countries, and many from eastern and southern Europe as well, found that the most commonly used antibiotics were penicillins, macrolides, and tetracyclines. The average per capita rate of consumption was 21.5 defined daily doses (DDD, equivalent to one day's treatment with an antibiotic) per 1,000 inhabitants. On average, antibiotic usage was lowest in northern European countries and higher in southern European countries. The Netherlands had the lowest consumption in 2012, at 11.3 DDD per 1,000, followed by Estonia (11.6 DDD per 1,000) and Latvia (13.1 DDD per 1,000). The highest use of antibiotics per capita was found in Greece (31.8 DDD per 1,000), followed by Romania (30.4 DDD per 1,000), and Belgium (29.8 DDD per 1,000).

WHAT IS ANTIMICROBIAL RESISTANCE?

Antimicrobial resistance means that an antimicrobial is not effective in killing a microorganism or inhibiting its growth. Some antimicrobial resistance is natural, in that not all antimicrobials are effective against all microorganisms, a phenomenon known as *natural* or *inherent resistance*. However, the term *antimicrobial resistance* is often reserved for acquired resistance, which refers to cases in which an antimicrobial that could previously kill or inhibit the growth of a microorganism is no longer effective against it. Antimicrobial resistance is a characteristic of the microorganism, not of the antimicrobial itself or of a person or animal being treated by the antimicrobial.

In medicine, some microbes are classified as being drug-resistant or multidrug-resistant. A *drug-resistant microbe* has become resistant to an antimicrobial that was previously effective against it. An example of a drug-resistant microbe is methicillin-resistant *Staphylococcus aureus* (MRSA), a type of staph bacteria that is resistant to methicillin, an antibiotic related to penicillin. A *multidrug-resistant microbe* is one that has become resistant to at least two drugs that were formerly effective against it. For instance, multidrug-resistant tuberculosis (MDR TB) is resistant to at least two common drugs used to treat TB: isoniazid and rifampin.

When common disease-causing microbes develop resistance to the drugs previously used against them, other drugs may be substituted. Drugs that are used in these instances are called *second-line drugs* because they are not the first drug of choice used in treating an infection but are used when the most common drug of choice (the first-line drug) is not effective. However, these other drugs may be less effective against the microbes or less desirable for other reasons: for instance, they may cause more side effects or be more expensive. Therefore, even if effective second-line drugs are available, the need to use them is a matter of public health concern because it raises the cost of treating infections and may bring about less satisfactory results. The development of drug-resistant and multidrug-resistant microbes is also a matter of public health because drug-resistant microbes may spread to other people, resulting in additional cases of disease that may be both more expensive and more difficult to treat satisfactorily.

How Microbes Become Resistant

A microbe may develop resistance to an antimicrobial drug in several ways, but the basis of all antimicrobial resistance is a basic principle of biology: selection pressure. The concept of selection pressure has no particular moral meaning; it simply refers to the observed phenomenon that in any population (whether microbes, insects, mammals, or some other life form), some members will be better equipped than others to respond to conditions in the environment and thus be more likely to survive and reproduce. *Selection pressure*, also known as *evolutionary pressure* and sometimes expressed colloquially as "survival of the fittest," refers to anything that favors individuals with certain inherited traits over those with other traits, and drug resistance is an excellent example of how selection pressure can shape a population.

In a given population of bacteria, most may be susceptible to a particular antibiotic, while a few may be resistant to it. If exposed to the drug (for instance, when a person takes penicillin to cure strep throat), the susceptible bacteria will be killed, while the resistant bacteria will survive. The surviving bacteria are then able to continue reproducing, while the susceptible bacteria are not. Over time, the population will contain a higher proportion of resistant bacteria. Although the proportion of resistant bacteria in a population may be very low to begin with, because bacteria populations grow quickly, a population may develop resistance to a specific antimicrobial surprisingly fast.

Mechanisms Producing Antimicrobial Resistance

Three biochemical mechanisms can produce antimicrobial resistance: mutation, destruction or inactivation, and efflux. In mutation, the DNA (the material that carries hereditary information in most organisms) of a microbe changes in a way that causes a change in the specific aspect of the microbe that makes it susceptible to an antimicrobial. When a microbe mutates in this way, the antimicrobial is no longer effective against it. The details of how mutation produces antimicrobial resistance are specific to the way a particular antimicrobial interacts with a specific microbe, but an example of this process may help to clarify the principle behind it. Fluoroquinolones, a class of antibiotics, bind with a specific enzyme, the DNA gyrase, within microbes, thus preventing them from replicating. If a microbe has a mutation that prevents a fluoroquinolone from binding with the microbe's DNA gyrase, then it is resistant to the drug and will not be killed by it. In this case, we would say that the microbe has developed resistance to fluoroquinolones.

In destruction or inactivation, the microbe has genes that produce enzymes to help the microbe resist an antimicrobial that would otherwise kill it. The enzymes produced by the microbe either degrade the antimicrobial so that it is no longer effective against the microbe or modify the antimicrobial so that it cannot reach and destroy its target within the microbe. In either case, the microbe has become resistant to the antimicrobial. In efflux, a pump mechanism within the microbe creates a channel that moves an antimicrobial that has entered the microbe out of it before the antimicrobial can accumulate in sufficient quantity to kill the microbe. In this case, the microbe also has become resistant to the antimicrobial.

Vertical and Horizontal Gene Transfer

A microbe that has developed genetic resistance to an antimicrobial can pass that trait on to its progeny (offspring), as is the case with other traits coded in DNA. This method of transmitting traits, including antimicrobial resistance, is known as *vertical gene transfer*. A second way that a microbe may acquire antimicrobial resistance is through *horizontal gene transfer*, also called *lateral gene transfer*. In horizontal gene transfer, genetic material is exchanged between existing microbes or between a dead microbe and a living one.

There are three mechanisms of horizontal gene transfer: conjugation, transformation, and transduction. *Conjugation* requires that two living microbes be in close proximity to each other and also requires the transfer of plasmids (a circular strand of DNA that can reproduce independently) from the cell that has resistance to the cell that does not; as a result of conjugation, the formerly susceptible microbe acquires resistance from the resistant microbe. In conjugation, a pilus, or hollow bridgelike structure, forms between the two microbes, and, as a plasmid is replicating, a copy is transferred from the resistant microbe to the nonresistant microbe. The formerly nonresistant microbe can thus acquire the same property of antimicrobial resistance as the resistant microbe.

Transformation takes place after cell death and breakdown (lysis). When a cell dies and breaks down, its genes (now called "naked" or free-floating DNA) can be transferred to other nearby cells, and these cells can incorporate the genes from the dead cell into their own DNA. In the case of microbes, when a resistant microbes dies and breaks down, neighboring cells may take in and incorporate the genes that made the dead cell resistant, acquiring antimicrobial resistance in this way.

In *transduction*, antibiotic resistance is acquired through infection with a virus that causes such resistance. Viruses reproduce by taking over the genetic processes of an infected cell, and when a virus moves from one cell to another, it may incorporate some of the DNA of the cell into its own DNA. When the cell dies and breaks up, this virus can infect other cells and transfer the resistance in this way.

WHY DRUG RESISTANCE IS A CONCERN

It is part of the normal process of evolution for microbes to become resistant to antimicrobials. However, when a microbe becomes resistant, that means that an antimicrobial is no longer effective in killing or limiting the growth of that microbe, so we have one less weapon to use in the fight against diseases that may be caused by that microbe. While modern science and medicine have many different antimicrobials that may be used against microbes, it is still a matter of serious concern every time one of the antimicrobials becomes ineffective.

Drug resistance will be discussed more thoroughly in the following chapters of this book. However, what is most important to remember is that the WHO has named drug resistance a serious threat to global public health because it diminishes our ability to prevent and treat a number of infections that can sicken or even kill people. Drug resistance has been identified throughout the world, and disease caused by a drug-resistant microbe can spread from one part of the world to another easily and quickly (for instance, when a person infected with the drug-resistant microbe takes a plane to travel from one continent to another).

Drug resistance affects our ability to treat many different types of diseases, including those caused by bacteria, such as TB, and those caused by parasites, such as malaria. When the usual or first-line treatments are not effective against diseases, physicians must use second- or third-line treatments, which may be more expensive, unavailable, or available only in limited quantities. As use of second- or third-line treatments increases, microbes will also develop resistance to them, so it will be necessary for new drugs to be developed in order to provide effective treatment against these microbes. If a microbe develops resistance to all the drugs available to treat it, the disease caused by the microbe is essentially untreatable. This is already close to happening with one common sexually transmitted disease, gonorrhea, as treatment failures have become increasingly common with all available drugs to treat it.

CHAPTER 2

The Role of Human Behavior in Drug Resistance

Antimicrobial resistance is a growing threat to human health, as more and more microbes become resistant to drugs that were formerly effective against them. In part, the development of antimicrobial resistance is part of the normal evolutionary process for microbes, as discussed in Chapter 1. However, human activity also plays a role in the development of antimicrobial resistance and may accelerate the process so that resistance develops much more quickly than it might otherwise. Two human activities play key roles in encouraging and accelerating the development of antimicrobial-resistant organisms: the inappropriate use of antimicrobials, and the use of low-quality antimicrobials.

INAPPROPRIATE USE OF DRUGS

Antimicrobials, including antibiotics, are important drugs that have saved millions of lives. However, they are not an appropriate treatment for every disease, and the inappropriate use of antimicrobials can hasten the development of microbes resistant to those drugs. Two types of inappropriate use are particularly relevant in fostering antimicrobial resistance: using antimicrobials to treat diseases for which they are not effective, and failing to take antimicrobials for the entire course of treatment prescribed. The first problem results in the overuse of antimicrobials, while the second results in their underuse. Both practices can foster the development of drug resistance in disease-causing microbes.

The overuse of antibiotics, particularly the use of antibiotics when they cannot possibly be effective, is one major factor encouraging the development of resistant microbes. Antibiotic overuse is common in many countries, both in the industrialized and developing worlds, and in rich and poor countries alike. In the United States and many other countries, antibiotics are available only by prescription. While theoretically the prescription requirement should ensure that antibiotics are used appropriately, in fact prescriptions are sometimes written to treat diseases for which antibiotics cannot be of use. For instance, common diseases such as colds, influenza, and many sore throats and ear infections are caused by viruses, and yet patients suffering from these conditions are sometimes prescribed antibiotics.

Prescription Antibiotics

In the United States, antibiotics are among the drugs most commonly prescribed for patients. While in many cases these prescriptions are appropriate and rational because an antibiotic is the appropriate treatment for a patient's condition, in other cases antibiotics are prescribed for conditions (such as viral infections) for which they are not effective. For instance, some studies have found that about 75 percent of antibiotics prescribed following physician visits (i.e., for an individual not in hospital care) are for conditions such as sinusitis, sore throat (pharyngitis), and bronchitis, which are commonly caused by viruses. Other studies have concluded that about half of all antibiotics prescribed during outpatient (as opposed to hospital) care are unnecessary. In addition, studies of the use of antibiotics in hospitals in the United States have found that the use of prescription antibiotics in some hospitals is three times as high as in other hospitals treating patients with similar conditions in similar parts of the hospital.

Inappropriate use of antibiotics has also been identified in other industrialized countries. In Europe, per capita use of antibiotics in some countries is three times as high as in other countries with similar disease profiles. For instance, in Greece in 2003, per capita outpatient use of antibiotics was about 30 defined daily doses (DDS), the amount of a drug typically used to treat one person for one day, per 1,000 population, while in the Netherlands, it was closer to 10 DDDs per 1,000. In general, antibiotic use is higher in Southern European countries than in Northern Europe. Because some researchers have identified an association between the level of antibiotic use in a country and the existence of drug-resistant strains of microbes, and because the resistant microbes can easily be transmitted to others both within the country and living in other countries, unusually high levels of use of antibiotics in particular countries is a global health concern.

In response to the overuse of prescription antibiotics, educational campaigns have been developed to inform both caregivers and patients about when antibiotics should and should not be used. For instance, the Centers for Disease Control and Prevention (CDC) in the United States created the "Get Smart: Know When Antibiotics Work" campaign to promote the effective use of antibiotics, with particular emphasis on the treatment of acute respiratory tract infections such as pharyngitis, sinusitis, and bronchitis. Evidence demonstrates that such campaigns can be effective in reducing the inappropriate use of prescription antibiotics. For instance, a study by Grace C. Lee and colleagues, published in *BMC Medicine* in 2014, showed that following the introduction of national educational campaigns about appropriate antibiotic use in the United States, overall antibiotic prescribing declined 18 percent for child and adolescent patients from 2000 to 2010.

France has an unusually high level of antibiotic use among European countries, with increased use during the winter season. In 2002, the National Health Insurance system in France launched a national campaign to decrease antibiotic use, with a particular focus on reducing the number of antibiotics prescribed to young children. Following this campaign, which used the slogan "Antibiotics are not automatic" to inform the public about the appropriate and inappropriate use of antibiotics, the use of prescription antibiotics per capita decreased by 26.5 percent over five years, as opposed to the two years before the campaign was launched. In addition, this campaign was followed by a 35.8 percent decrease in antibiotic use per capita among children aged 6 through 15 years.

Australia also conducted a successful campaign to reduce the number of antibiotics prescribed nationally. In 1998, the National Prescribing Service was created to further the appropriate use of medicines. This campaign had multiple components, including professional education and consumer awareness strategies, as well as a National Prescribing Curriculum for medical and pharmacy students. This curriculum emphasized the appropriate and inappropriate use of antibiotics in health care. During and after the campaign, the overall number of antibiotics prescribed in Australia fell from 15.5 prescriptions per 100 medical encounters in 1999 to 13.25 per 100 encounters in 2007. In addition, the number of prescriptions for antibiotics commonly used to treat upper respiratory tract infections fell from 80 per 1,000 consultations in 1996 to 50 per 1,000 consultations in 2007.

Antibiotics Without a Prescription

Antibiotics are available without a prescription in many countries, and globally, about two-thirds of antibiotics are sold without a prescription. Even in countries like the United States, where theoretically the purchase of antibiotics requires a prescription, antibiotics are sometimes available without a prescription through means such as Internet sales. Dispensing antibiotics without a prescription has also been noted to occur in European countries where the practice is forbidden by law.

The greater problem, however, is in countries where antibiotic drugs are customarily dispensed from pharmacies and other sources with no expectation that the purchaser obtain a prescription first. The sale of antibiotics without a prescription is worrying because it often results in the overuse of antibiotics and their use for conditions not responsive to antibiotics, such as viral infections. In general, the increased use of antibiotics creates the conditions for faster development of resistant strains of bacteria. Also, the use of antibiotics for conditions for which they are ineffective does not help the ill person, but it does promote the growth of resistant strains of bacteria, increasing the probability that in the future, people will become infected with resistant strains of bacteria that do not respond to the usual drug treatments.

Particularly among the poor and those living in poor countries, the inappropriate use of antibiotics may be a decision encouraged or forced by financial circumstances. This is especially true in developing countries that lack an inadequate infrastructure to provide even basic health services to all members of the population. The problem begins with lack of access to proper diagnostic services, as a poor individual may not be able to pay the consultation fees and may live far from a qualified practitioner. The individual also may not be able to purchase enough drugs to follow a full course of treatment, so that purchasing enough for a partial regimen may be the only available choice. In addition, the choice of drug may be affected by cost, so the individual chooses the cheapest, rather than the most appropriate, drug, even if the cheapest drug may not be ideal (or even effective at all) for treating the illness in question.

In many countries, unofficial sources of drugs, including antibiotics, exist alongside the official system. A person who cannot afford the time and expense of seeking a diagnosis from a qualified practitioner and purchasing an adequate supply of an effective drug from a source of guaranteed quality may purchase cheap antibiotics from one of these unofficial sources. The result may be not only that the medicine is ineffective against the illness, but also that its use furthers the development of antibiotic resistance.

Treatment Adherence

Worldwide, patient adherence to treatment regimens is estimated at approximately 50 percent, with less adherence in developing countries. Treatment adherence is particularly important with antibiotics and other antimicrobials. This is because a patient treated with an antibiotic may feel better early in the course of treatment due to reduced pathogen load (i.e., the drug has killed many of the microorganisms causing the disease), but still has pathogens in his or her body. If the full course of treatment is not followed, the remaining pathogens, including those with some resistance to the antibiotic, will not be killed. Instead, they will be able to reproduce, and their survival will not be threatened by the antibiotic. Under these conditions, the disease may recur in the patient, requiring a further course of treatment. In addition, the partial exposure to antibiotics favors the survival of resistant strains of the pathogen due to selective pressure, thus creating the potential for greater problems with drug resistance in the future.

USE OF LOW-QUALITY DRUGS

Another source of antimicrobial resistance is use of low-quality drugs. Antibiotics and other antimicrobials are normally prescribed in a strength that is sufficient to kill the target pathogen, if the drug is taken as specified and for the full course of treatment. When the drug supplied is of lower strength than specified, the antibiotics may kill some of (but not all) the microbes, with those that have resistance to the microbe being favored, or selected, for survival. This process not only endangers the health of the individual taking the drug (because the infection may not be completely cured), but also endangers the health of the overall population by encouraging the survival and reproduction of resistant microbes.

The use of drugs that do not contain the specified quantity of their active ingredients is not a major problem in the United States and other developed countries. However, in developing countries in particular, insufficient regulation and quality assurance means that people prescribed antibiotics may be supplied with medication that is not strong enough to completely kill the microbes causing the disease. For the most part, the problem is not one of individual choices on the part of either the patient or the physician, but of inadequate regulation of the medicine supply, the manufacturing process, or both. It may also be a problem of economics, in that an individual may not be able to afford high-quality medicine and thus purchases or otherwise obtains a low-quality medicine to treat an illness. A third possibility is fraud, in which a counterfeit medicine that does not contain the specified active ingredient or does not contain the level of the specified ingredient is supplied and sold as if it were a legitimate, therapeutic-quality medicine. A fourth possibility is that of the use of expired or spoiled medicine due to the unavailability of current, high-quality medicine and breakdowns in the supply chain so that good medicines are spoiled due to improper storage or other issues.

Problems with low-quality drugs are most common in countries with poor infrastructure in the healthcare sector. Often, these countries do not have a national system of quality control or comprehensive legislation covering all aspects of the pharmaceutical industry. Even if adequate regulations exist, they may be poorly implemented due to lack of resources, corruption, or other reasons. Even within a well-planned system of drug procurement, storage, and distribution, quality control may fail due to faulty execution at some point of the process, so high-quality drugs are inadequately supplied to some area of the country or good drugs may be spoiled due to poor storage conditions or expiration.

In a country where the distribution system for medicines is inadequate, people living in rural areas may have less access to effective, high-quality drugs than people living in cities. The lack of access to drugs compounds the effects of two facts about infectious disease in the modern world: poor countries bear most of the burden of infectious disease, and the poorest people within those countries bear a disproportionate share of that burden. The poor, and people living in poor countries, are thus most likely both to suffer from an infection requiring medical treatment and to lack access to drugs adequate to treating that infection.

USE OF ANTIMICROBIALS IN ANIMAL HUSBANDRY

In animal husbandry, antibiotics may be used as growth promoters for food animals (e.g., cattle, poultry, and hogs), as prophylactic treatments (to prevent disease in healthy animals), and to treat specific infections or illnesses. The third use of antibiotics, to treat diseased animals, is not controversial, but the first and second uses of antibiotics are. The controversial use of antibiotics in animal husbandry is described in more detail in Chapter 11.

CHAPTER 3

The Scope of the Problem Today

Drug resistance is a global problem that is expected to increase in the coming years. In part, this is because drug resistance is a natural phenomenon. As explained in Chapter 1, it is part of the normal process of evolution for any microbe to develop resistance to substances that formerly could kill it or inhibit its growth. Increased use of antimicrobials worldwide can therefore be expected to result in the increased development of antimicrobial-resistant organisms. This is one of the paradoxes of antimicrobial use: While antimicrobials are extremely useful drugs that can both save lives and improve the quality of life, their use also can lead to them becoming ineffective.

Although antimicrobial resistance is an expected result of antimicrobial use, there are many things that people can do to limit or lessen this problem, and these measures will be discussed further in Chapter 5. However, an important step in understanding the problem of antimicrobial resistance is becoming aware of the scope of the problem, and the purpose of this chapter is to describe the extent of antimicrobial resistance, both globally and in the United States.

GLOBAL OVERVIEW OF DRUG RESISTANCE

According to the World Health Organization (WHO), antimicrobial resistance is a growing threat to public health around the world. While the 20th century was characterized by a dramatic reduction in the threat of many previously common, sometimes life-threatening diseases thanks to the development of antibiotics and other antimicrobial drugs, the growing threat of antimicrobial resistance threatens to place the world in a postantibiotic era in which no effective treatment is available for the most common infectious diseases and where even a minor break in the skin may become life-threatening due to infection.

Measuring any problem on a worldwide basis presents challenges, and antimicrobial resistance is no different. The extent and quality of antimicrobial resistance surveillance vary from one country to the next, and even within a single country, the surveillance process may not be well coordinated. However, even imperfect information can help estimate the extent of a problem and aid in crafting responses to it.

Antibacterial Resistance

As part of the effort to combat antimicrobial resistance worldwide, the WHO produced a global report on the topic in 2014. This report focused primarily on antibacterial resistance in common disease-causing bacteria because bacteria cause some of the most common, and potentially deadliest, diseases in both humans and animals. This report is the primary resource for global information about antibacterial resistance.

The key conclusions from the WHO report are disturbing. It indicates that many common pathogens (disease-causing organisms) associated with diseases contracted in healthcare settings (e.g., hospitals or physician's offices), such as pneumonia and URIs (upper respiratory tract infections), have high rates of resistance to the drugs commonly used to treat them. In addition, these high rates of resistance have been found in all WHO regions (namely, Africa, the Americas, South-East Asia, Europe, the Eastern Mediterranean, and the Western Pacific). Finally, the WHO concludes that, due to gaps in reporting, particularly from the less-developed countries of the world, the problem of antimicrobial resistance is probably worse than currently realized.

The WHO report focuses on seven common types of bacteria that cause human disease. Three of these bacteria are associated with infections acquired in both hospitals and the community (for instance, in private households or in schools): *Escherichia coli* (*E. coli*), and *Staphylococcus aureus* (*S. aureus*). Four of the bacteria studied are associated with infections in the community: namely, *Streptococcus pneumoniae*, nontyphoidal *Salmonella*, *Shigella*, and *Neisseria gonorrhea*. Reports of high levels of resistance (50 percent or more for pathogens associated with hospital-acquired infections, and 25 percent or more for pathogens associated with both hospital- and community-acquired infections) are collected from national reports, and the number of WHO regions in which high levels of resistance is tallied to give an idea of the global extent of drug resistance for each pathogen.

E. coli is a type of bacteria that commonly exists in the lower intestine of some warm-blooded mammals, including humans and cattle, and in fecal matter. There are many strains of *E. coli*, and most are harmless, with some in fact being necessary for good health (e.g., they help create some vitamins during the digestive process). However, a few strains can cause serious disease and even death. Some strains of *E. coli* produce Shiga toxin, which can produce severe, bloody diarrhea and kidney failure in humans. Other strains of *E. coli* can cause serious URIs and bloodstream infections, and it is these strains that are of the greatest concern for global public health. *E. coli* is the most frequent cause of URIs in both hospital and community settings, the most frequent cause of bloodstream infections, and a leading cause of foodborne illness.

While the *E. coli* strains causing bloodstream and URIs are commonly treated by antibiotics in the fluoroquinolones and third-generation celphalosporin classes, they are increasingly becoming resistant to these drugs. As of 2014, countries in five of the six WHO regions reported finding that at least half of *E. coli* infections were resistant to fluoroquinolones and third-generation cephalosporins. While a different class of antibacterial, *carbapenems*, is still useful in treating resistant *E. coli*, those drugs are more expensive and less available, making treatment particularly difficult in low-income countries.

Klebsiella pneumoniae is a type of bacteria that can cause many different types of disease, including pneumonia, meningitis, wound infections, bloodstream infections, and URIs. *Klebsiella* bacteria are normally found in the human intestines (although they do not cause disease in that location) and are also found in human fecal matter. However, when introduced into other parts of the body, including the bloodstream, urinary tract, and respiratory tract, *Klebsiella* bacteria can cause serious illness. *Klebsiella* infection is most commonly found among people being treated in hospitals, particularly those who are seriously ill, are taking certain types of antibiotics, or require the use of a ventilator (breathing machine) or an intravenous catheter (a tube inserted into a vein). While *Klebsiella* infections have been treated successfully with third-generation cephalosporins, some countries in all six WHO regions have reported at least 50 percent resistance to this usual mode of treatment. In addition, countries in two of the six WHO regions report at least 50 percent resistance to treatment with third-generation carbapenems.

S. aureus is a type of bacteria in the *Staphylococcus* or staph family. Staph bacteria are extremely numerous and are commonly found on the skin and in the noses of many people, even in healthy individuals. However, if staph bacteria enter a wound, the result can be a serious infection. Staph bacteria played a key role in the discovery of the first broad-spectrum anti-biotic, penicillin, when Alexander Fleming discovered that a spot of mold in a petri dish apparently had the ability to kill the staph bacteria in the dish. Staph infections were successfully treated with antibiotics for years, but some types of staph have become resistance to some commonly used anti-biotics. One of those strains is methicillin-resistant *S. aureus* (MRSA), which (as you might guess from the name) is resistant to methicillin, an antibiotic in the penicillin class. MRSA infections are contracted most often in hospitals and other healthcare facilities and are particularly common among individuals who have devices such as intravenous lines or urinary catheters inserted into their bodies. As of 2014, countries in five of the six WHO regions reported at least 50 percent of *S. aureus* infections were resis-tant to methicillin. While other drugs are available to treat *S. aureus* infec-tions, they are generally more expensive and have more severe side effects than the first-line treatments.

S. pneumoniae is a bacteria in the *Streptococcus* or strep family. As the name indicates, *S. pneumoniae* can cause pneumonia, but it is also associ-ated with other types of infections, including meningitis (inflammation of the membranes around the brain and spinal cord) and otitis (ear infections). Countries in all six WHO regions report finding strains of *S. pneumoniae* resistant or nonsusceptible to penicillin in at least 25 percent of cases, and some report over 50 percent of cases feature resistant strains.

Salmonella is a type of bacteria that has over 2,500 serotypes (distinct groupings based on surface structures), with some found in only one part of the world or infecting only one type of animal. While it is not completely known which types of *Salmonella* pose a threat to human health, fewer than 100 serotypes of salmonella are believed to be able to infect people. One type of salmonella that is particularly relevant to public health is *nontyphoi-dal Salmonella*, which can cause a common type of food poisoning, salmo-nellosis, as well as bloodstream infections. Globally, tens of millions of people each year are sickened by salmonellosis, usually through food poi-soning, and although most cases of food poisoning are mild, some are fatal. Since the 1990s, increasing salmonella resistance to antimicrobials has been observed, and in 2014, countries in three of the six WHO regions reported at least 25 percent of nontyphoidal *Salmonella* strains were resis-tant to fluoroquinolones. In addition to the difficulties posed in treating infections, the development of resistant strains of salmonella is a health con-cern because these new strains are associated with worse patient outcomes.

Shigella is a type of bacteria spread through fecal matter that is closely related to salmonella that can cause severe diarrhea and dysentery (diarrhea with blood and mucus in the stools), fever, abdominal cramps, and mucosal ulceration (open sores in the mucous membranes lining the intestines). *Shigella* is spread by consumption of contaminated food or water, but it can also be transmitted through swimming in contaminated water or by direct contact with the bacteria. Most *Shigella* infection can be treated with fluoroquinolones, but as of 2014, countries in two of the six WHO regions reported at least 25 percent resistance of *Shigella* to this type of antibiotic. Rates of drug-resistant *Shigella* may be even higher than reported because surveillance is poor in some of the countries with the highest rates of disease caused by this organism. In addition, drug-resistant strains of this pathogen have been associated with more serious cases of disease than earlier strains.

N. gonorrhea is a species of bacteria that causes gonorrhea, a sexually transmitted disease that can cause many health threats, including infertility and neonatal eye infections (i.e., eye infection at birth) leading to blindness, and is also associated with increased risk of HIV transmission. Gonorrhea is a common disease worldwide, with about 88 million new cases annually, and is theoretically curable with antibiotics. However, *N. gonorrhea* began showing resistance to antibiotics almost as soon as they were first used to treat it, and it currently has such high rates of resistance to several classes of antibiotics, including penicillin, tetracycline, macrolides, sulfonamides, and quinolone, that these medications are no longer recommended for treating it. The current treatment of choice for gonorrhea is third-generation cephalospirins, but increasing rates of resistance suggest that soon this type of antibiotic may also become ineffective, leaving medicine with no effective treatment for this disease. As of 2014, countries in three of the six WHO regions reported at least 25 percent of *N. gonorrhea* cases were resistant to third-generation cehalosporins. Because surveillance for drug-resistant gonorrhea is poor in some of the countries with the highest rates of infection, the spread of drug-resistant strains of this disease may be even higher than reported.

Drug Resistance for Specific Diseases

Specific diseases in which drug resistance is a public health problem are discussed in Chapter 4, but a brief overview of a few major diseases in this category helps create a context for this chapter.

One of the most-publicized drug-resistant diseases, in part because several cases in the United States received extensive news coverage, is tuberculosis (TB). However, the problem of drug-resistant TB and multidrug-resistant TB (MDR TB) is global, with the highest rates of occurrence in Eastern Europe and Central Asia. Globally, 3.6 percent of new TB cases annually are MDR TB, as are 20.2 percent of previously treated cases.

Because MDR TB does not respond to the drugs that previously were effective against TB, it is much more difficult to cure, and the treatment success rate is lower. For instance, among patients that began treatment in 2010, fewer than half (48 percent) were cured following completion of treatment. Treatment success rates are even lower for those with extensively drug-resistant TB (XDR TB). The low success rate for curing people infected with MDR TB and XDR TB means that there is an increasing population of people still infected with these diseases, who thus can spread them to others.

The introduction of antiretroviral drugs to treat HIV infection and AIDS was one of the great medical breakthroughs of the late 20th century. Advances in the treatment of HIV infection and AIDS have changed these conditions from a certain death sentence to long-term, chronic diseases. However, like all bacteria, viruses have the ability to become resistant to drugs that formerly were effective in killing them or limiting their growth. Studies of people beginning antiretroviral treatment for HIV infection or AIDS increasingly reveal that many are infected with drug-resistant strains of the virus. Outcomes are expected to be poorer for these individuals because drug-resistant strains of HIV are more likely to survive treatment with the usual drugs, and hence viral replication will proceed and the disease will progress rather than being suppressed. Several studies suggest that in Australia, Europe, Japan, and the United States, among those infected with HIV who that have not previously been treated with antiretrovirals, 10 to 17 percent are infected with HIV strains that are resistant to at least one antiretroviral drug.

Influenza (flu) is a common respiratory illness caused by a number of related viruses. Flu is highly contagious, and although in most years, most cases of flu are mild and self-limiting, there are cases of flu every year that result in severe complications and death. In addition, some strains of flu are more severe than others, and the world has experienced several flu pandemics (disease outbreaks across much of the world) with high levels of infection and death. Vaccines and antiviral drugs have been developed to help reduce the incidence of flu and to lessen the severity of the disease for those already infected. However, resistance to some commonly used flu drugs, including adamantine antivirals and oseltamivir (sold under the brand name Tamiflu), has been reported, suggesting that the effectiveness of these drugs may already be reduced.

Antimalarial Drug Resistance

Malaria is a preventable and curable disease transmitted to humans through the bite of a mosquito infected with *Plasmodium*, the parasite that causes the disease. A person infected with malaria typically experiences fever, chills, anemia, and flulike symptoms, and it is a particular threat to pregnant women and small children. This disease has been a significant threat to human health for centuries and remains so in many parts of the world, most commonly in developing countries. The significance of malaria to human health, as well as the difficulty in finding ways to control and treat it, are evident from the fact that the Nobel Prize in Physiology or Medicine has been awarded four times to researchers studying malaria: in 1902, to Sir Ronald Ross; in 1907, to Louise Alphonse Laveran; in 1927, to Julius Wagner-Jauregg; and in 1948, to Paul Hermann Müller.

Although malaria is rare in the United States today (there are about 1,500 to 2,000 cases reported each year, almost all associated with foreign travel), this was not always the case. In fact, the predecessor organization for the Centers for Disease Control and Prevention (CDC) was the Office of Malaria Control in War Areas, founded in 1942. Efforts to prevent and control malaria were so successful that by 1949, malaria was no longer a significant public health threat in the United States.

Globally, about half the world's population is at risk for malaria, and in 2014, malaria transmission was ongoing in 97 countries and territories in the world. In 2013, there were about 198 million cases of malaria globally, with an estimated 584,000 deaths. Children in Africa are at the greatest risk of death from malaria. Malaria prevention and treatment efforts have greatly reduced the burden of disease and death from malaria, with an estimated 47 percent reduction in malaria mortality rates and an estimated 58 percent reduction in malaria mortality rates among children in Africa between 2000 and 2013. Prevention measures for malaria include removing the breeding grounds for mosquitoes, spraying with insecticide, and using bed nets (made of fine mesh, sometimes treated with insecticide) to create a screen around a bed so the mosquitoes cannot reach people and bite them while they sleep). Treatment for malaria typically includes the administration of several different types of drugs to reduce symptoms and kill the parasites that cause the disease.

Malaria is spread through the bite of *Anopheles* mosquitoes, which mainly attack between dusk and dawn (hence the importance of using bed nets to prevent infection). The mosquitoes breed in still water (hence the importance of removing breeding grounds by actions such as draining swamps or spraying sources of standing water with insecticide). Four parasite species cause malaria in humans: *Plasmodium falciparum*, *Plasmodium vivax*, *Plasmodium malariae*, and *Plasmodium ovale*. The most common species are *P. falciparum* and *P. vivax*, while *P. falciparum* is the species deadliest to humans. A person can be infected with malaria, survive, and develop immunity to it; most deaths due to malaria occur in young children who have not had time to develop immunity.

Early diagnosis and treatment are key to lessening the severity of malaria, preventing death, and reducing transmission. Several methods are available to confirm a case of malaria, with results available in approximately 15 minutes. Treatment on the basis of symptoms alone is not recommended, however, because the symptoms can resemble those of many other diseases, particularly in the early stages of malaria. The best available treatment for malaria is artemisinin-based combination therapy (ACT), which provides effective treatment while limiting the development of drug-resistant *Plasmodium* parasites. ACT replaces several drugs formerly used to treat malaria, including chloroquine and sulfadoxine plus pyrimethamine (brand name Fansidar), because the *Plamodium* parasite developed resistance to those drugs.

Artemisinin is a drug derived from the sweet wormwood (*Artemisia annua* or *Qing hao*) plant, which is also used to treat malaria in Chinese traditional medicine. Artemisinin causes a quick reduction of the number of parasites in the bloodstream, providing the infected individual with symptomatic relief. However, this treatment does not completely kill the parasites in the person's body, so the disease can recur. This scenario, in which some but not all parasites are killed, also creates ideal conditions for the creation of parasites resistant to artemisinin, threatening the future effectiveness of this drug as an antimalarial.

For this reason, the WHO does not recommend the use of artemisinin alone (monotherapy) to treat malaria; instead, it recommends that the drug be used in combination with other drugs, such as mefloquine or lumefantrine. The use of these combination drugs provides superior results for the infected individual, lessens the risk of developing drug-resistant parasites, and reduces the probability of the infected person passing the *Plasmodium* parasite to mosquitoes that can then infect other people. Cases of malaria resistant to artemisinin has already been reported in the southeastern Asia countries of Cambodia, Laos, Myanmar, Thailand, and Vietnam, and if this resistance spreads, it could create a global health crisis by making the most common antimalarial drug ineffective in treating the disease and slowing its spread.

A second problem of drug resistance related to malaria is that of mosquitoes developing resistance to the insecticides used to kill them. Indoor residual spraying (IRS), in which insecticide is applied to the indoor surfaces of dwellings (e.g., walls) where mosquitoes may rest, is one method used to contain mosquitoes and thus lessen the spread of malaria. IRS is most effective when at least 80 percent of homes in a targeted area are sprayed. The insecticides currently recommended for IRS contain pyre-throids, organic compounds that repel insects but are not harmful to humans in low doses. However, mosquito resistance to pyrethroids has been detected in some countries, with widespread reports of resistance in some parts of India and sub-Saharan Africa that are also characterized by high rates of malaria transmission.

Health and Economic Burden of Antibacterial Resistance

Drug resistance creates a burden for individuals and countries in terms of both health (e.g., a more serious case of the disease, slower recovery from the disease, or higher death rates) and economics (e.g., lost income and productivity). Looking first at health, the WHO studied differences in out-comes due to drug resistance for three microbes: *E. coli*, *K. pneumoniae*, and *S. aureus*.

Patients infected with cephalosporin-resistant *E. coli* had a twofold increase in mortality compared to those infected with nonresistant *E. coli*; these statistics included all-cause mortality (death from any cause), bacterium-attributable mortality (death due to infection with the bacteria), and 30-day mortality (death within 30 days of diagnosis with the infection). However, individuals infected with cephalosporin-resistant *E. coli* did not experience an increased length of stay (LOS) in the hospital (i.e., they did not spend more days in the hospital on average) or increased admission to an intensive care unit (ICU), as compared to those infected with nonresis-tant *E. coli*. Patients infected with fluoroquinolone-resistant *E. coli* had a twofold increase in all-cause mortality and 30-day mortality, but no sig-nificant increase in bacterium-attributable morality or LOS, compared to those infected with nonresistant *E. coli*. Those infected with fluoroquinolone-resistant *E. coli* also showed an increased risk of ICU admission or septic shock (a life-threatening condition caused by infection and characterized by very low blood pressure).

Patients infected with *K. pneumoniae* resistant to third-generation ceph-alosporins, as compared to those infected with nonresistant *K. pneumonia*, were at an increased risk of ICU admission, all-cause mortality, bacterium-attributable mortality, and 30-day mortality. However, they were not at significantly greater risk for increased LOS or septic shock. Patients infected with *K. pneumoniae* resistant to carbapanems were at greater risk for all-cause mortality and 30-day mortality, but not bacterium-attributable mor-tality or increased LOS.

Patients infected with MRSA, as opposed to nonresistant strains of *S. aureus*, were at significantly greater risk for all-cause mortality, bacterium-attributable mortality, septic shock, ICU mortality (dying in the ICU), and increased postinfection LOS (increased time in the hospital following infection). They were also at increased risk to discharge to long-term care facilities. However, they were not at greater risk of 30-day mortality, overall increased LOS, or ICU admission.

Unfortunately, there are large gaps in our knowledge regarding the economic burden imposed by infection with drug-resistant pathogens. Most studies addressing this question have been conducted in countries classified by the World Bank as upper-middle or high income, based on per capita gross national income (GNI), while relatively fewer studies have been conducted in countries classified as low or lower-middle income. In addition, available information is primarily limited to costs imposed on the healthcare system rather than the more general question of economic burden, including issues such as lost productivity due to illness or premature mortality. In addition, relatively few studies have been conducted to date, and differences in design among studies (for instance, the comparison group for subjects infected with drug-resistant pathogens might be uninfected persons in one study and those infected with nonresistant strains of the same pathogen in another), make general conclusions difficult.

However, several studies have addressed the economic effects of drug-resistant infections from *E. coli* and MRSA. Infection with *E. coli* resistant to third-generation cephalosporins is associated with increased costs due to hospitalization, antibacterial therapy (including cost of medication, monitoring, and adverse event management), and overall medical care. It should be noted that these results were based on a relatively small sample of one or two studies per cost category. More research has been devoted to quantifying the increased costs of infection with MRSA (up to 17 studies per cost category), and these studies found that MRSA is associated with increased costs due to hospitalization, antibacterial therapy, and overall medical care.

Drug Resistance in the United States

The CDC estimates that over 2 million people each year in the United States become ill from infections from antimicrobial-resistant pathogens, with about 23,000 dying from such infections. Antibiotic-resistant infections also raise healthcare costs due to extended hospital stays, longer or costlier treatments, additional physician visits, and greater disability and death. In 2013, the CDC estimated that antimicrobial resistance costs the U.S. healthcare system $20 billion per year, and that costs due to lost productivity due to antimicrobial resistance may be as high as $35 billion annually. In addition, infection with the bacteria *Clostridium difficile* (*C. difficile*), which is not itself antibiotic resistant but is linked to the use of antibiotics and exposure to other resistant pathogens, is estimated to cause at least 250,000 illnesses and 14,000 deaths annually.

The CDC classifies disease-causing pathogens into three categories, depending on the degree to which their resistance to antibiotics poses a health concern in the United States. Factors included in making these classifications include clinical and economic impact, current and projected 10-year incidence (the number of new cases recorded each year and expected over the next 10 years), transmissibility, availability of effective treatments, and barriers to prevention. A total of 12 pathogens are classified as serious threats, and 3 as concerning threats. The highest level of threat, urgent, is reserved for 3 pathogens: *C. difficile*, carbapenem-resistant *Enterobacteriaceae* (CRE), and drug-resistant *N. gonorrhoeae*.

Urgent Threats

Three antimicrobial-resistant pathogens are classified as urgent threats because they pose significant risks with potentially high consequences. Although infection from these pathogens may not be widespread currently, they have the potential to cause widespread attention and thus require action from the public health sphere to identify infections and limit their transmission.

C. difficile is a bacteria that causes an estimated 250,000 infections and 14,000 deaths annually in the United States, as well as an estimated $1 billion in excess medical costs. *C. difficile* infections occur most commonly in people taking antibiotics, including those who are hospitalized or have recently been hospitalized; people currently living in a nursing home; and people who have recently visited a clinic or physician's office for care. *C. difficile* infection can cause severe diarrhea, which can lead to death, particularly for elderly people; although just over half of these infections occur in people over 65, over 90 percent of the deaths due to *C. difficile* occur in that age group.

C. difficile is a particular threat to human health today due to the emergence of a stronger strain of this bacteria around 2000, and the United States saw a 400 percent increase in deaths related to this infection between 2000 and 2007. This strain of *C. difficile* bacteria is resistant to fluoroquinolones, a type of antibiotics used to treat other infections. This highlights a particular concern with treating it: although this bacteria has not yet developed resistance to the drugs used to combat it, it is naturally resistant to many of the antibiotics commonly used to treat other infections.

CRE is responsible for an estimated 9,300 drug-resistant infections annually in the United States, as well as about 600 deaths. Infection with CRE is associated with receiving care in medical facilities, including hospitals. Annually, about 140,000 cases of infection with *Enterobacteriaceae* are identified in the United States, and although carbapenem-resistant infections are currently only a small fraction of those cases, this percentage is growing. In addition, CRE is generally resistant to nearly all other antibiotics, with the carbapenem class being the treatment of last resort; therefore, there are few to no effective treatment options for those infected with CRE.

The presence of CRE is a widespread problem, with the CDC reporting that at least one healthcare facility in 44 of the 50 U.S. states has had at least one confirmed case of CRE (the lack of such cases in the other 6 states could be due either to the fact that CRE is not present, or that it is present but not detected). CRE is more common in long-term, acute care hospitals (it has been identified in 18 percent of hospitals of this type) than in short-stay hospitals (where it has been identified in 4 percent of hospitals of this type). Although bloodstream infections with CRE are relatively rare, they are also serious, with about half of patients with CRE bloodstream infections dying as a result of the infection.

As noted earlier, *N. gonorrhoeae* causes the sexually transmitted disease gonorrhea. Gonorrhea is a common disease in the United States, being the second most commonly reported notifiable infection (i.e., a disease that must be reported to the government). It is readily transmitted through unprotected sexual activity. About 820,000 cases of gonorrhea are reported each year in the United States, of which about 246,000 (30 percent) are resistant to one or more antibiotics normally used to treat this disease. Although rarely fatal, untreated gonorrhea can cause pelvic inflammatory disease in women, a condition associated with sterility and long-term abdominal pain, and it is also associated with a higher probability of transmitting or becoming infected with HIV, which causes AIDS, a potentially fatal disease.

The CDC estimates that 30 percent of cases of gonorrhea in the United States are caused by a strain of *N. gonorrhoeae* that is resistant to at least one antibiotic. The most common type of resistance, found in about 23 percent of cases, is to tetracyclines. Other types of resistance are rarer, accounting for less than 1 percent of cases, and include resistance to cefixime (an oral type of cephalosporin), ceftriaxone (an injectable type of cephalosporin), and azithromycin. Because gonorrhea is a common disease and is easily spread, the emergence of a strain resistant to cephalosporins, a type of antibiotic currently used to treat this disease, makes treating and controlling this disease more difficult and complicated. This is particularly true because strains resistant to cephalosporins are often resistant to other antibiotics as well. Finally, the presence of drug-resistant gonorrhea limits one important means of preventing the spread of gonorrhea (namely, reducing the number of infected people in the population, so that fewer people are exposed to the disease) because this strategy depends on the availability of reliable, effective treatments.

Serious Threats

The CDC has classified 12 pathogens as serious threats, with the understanding that any of them could progress to the level of an urgent threat if adequate public health response is not forthcoming. Serious threats differ from urgent threats in that the incidence of infections from these threats may be low or declining, or there may currently be adequate treatments for disease caused by these pathogens. However, effective monitoring and prevention programs are required to prevent these threats from worsening.

Acinetobacter is a type of bacteria that can cause pneumonia and bloodstream infections, most commonly in critically ill patients, with infection frequently occurring in a healthcare context. About 12,000 infections and 500 deaths are caused annually by *Acinetobacter* in the United States. Almost two-thirds (63 percent) of *Acinetobacter* strains are MDR, meaning that they are resistant to at least three classes of antibiotics that had been effective against them. Some strains are resistant to all antibiotics currently used against them, including carbapenems, which are considered a treatment of last resort for drug-resistant bacterial infections.

Campylobacter is a type of bacteria that can cause severe diarrhea, fever, and abdominal cramping and is sometimes associated with more serious conditions, such as temporary paralysis. Infection with *Campylobacter* is quite common, occurring about 1.3 million times per year in the United States, with 13,000 cases requiring hospitalization and 120 resulting in death. Drug resistance to *Campylobacter* increased from 13 percent in 1997 to 25 percent in 2011, with almost 25 percent of strains showing resistance to ciprofloxacin, 2 percent showing resistance to azithromycin, and 24 percent showing resistance to both azithromycin and ciprofloxacin.

Candida is a type of fungus that is normally present in the mucous membranes (including the mouth and intestinal tract) and on the skin of humans. However, over 20 species of *Candida* can infect humans, and overgrowth of *Candida* can cause illness, with the greatest risk to people who are already seriously ill or have suppressed immune systems. The most common type of *Candida* potentially dangerous to humans is *Candida albicans*, which poses a significant risk to people with compromised immune systems, including those with AIDS, those who are receiving chemotherapy, or those who are undergoing a bone marrow transplant. *Candida* is the fourth-most-common cause of healthcare-related infections, with an estimated 46,000 infections annually and 220 deaths. The growth of drug-resistant strains of

Candida (7 percent of infections are resistant to flucanazoles) is particularly worrying because of the potentially severe consequences to infected patients: For instance, about 30 percent of patients with drug-resistant bloodstream *Candida* infections die as a result of the infection. In addition, the CDC estimates that treatment for drug-resistant strains of *Candida* results in millions of dollars of additional healthcare costs in the United States each year.

Enterobacteriaceae are a class of bacteria that includes many familiar types of disease-causing bacteria, including *Salmonella*, *E. coli*, *Shigella*, *Klebsiella*, and *Yersinia pestis* (the cause of plague). An estimated 140,000 infections caused by *Enterobacteriaceae* occur in healthcare settings annually in the United States, with 1,700 resulting in death. The emergence of strains of *Enterobacteriaceae* resistant to extended-spectrum β-lactamase (ESBL) antibiotics, a class of antibiotics that includes the penicillins and cephalosporins, represents a serious health threat, with about 28 percent of healthcare-related *Enterobacteriaceae* infections being resistant to ESBL antibiotics. While these infections can be treated successfully by carbapanems, a different class of antibiotics, increased use of carbapanems ultimately results in the bacteria being resistant to them as well.

Enterococci are a type of bacteria that can cause many illnesses, including URIs, bloodstream and surgical site infections, endocarditis (inflammation of the inner tissues of the heart), and meningitis. About 66,000 infections from *Enterococci* occur in healthcare settings each year, resulting in about 1,300 deaths. About 30.3 percent of infections with *Enterococci* are resistant to vancomycin, an antibiotic used as a treatment of last resort; there are currently no effective antibiotic treatments for infections caused by these resistant strains of *Enterococci* .

Pseudomonas aeruginosa is a type of bacteria commonly found on the skin and in the environment but that also can cause disease in humans, particularly those with weakened immune systems. *P. aeruginosa* is a common cause of healthcare-related infections, including pneumonia, URIs, surgical site infections, and bloodstream infections. About 51,000 infections with *P. aeruginosa* occur each year, and 440 deaths. About 13 percent of *P. aeruginosa* infections are caused by MDR strains (meaning they are resistant to several different classes of antibiotics), with some strains resistant to all or nearly all currently available antibiotics.

Nontyphoidal Salmonella (varieties of *Salmonella* that do not cause typhoid fever) can cause bloody diarrhea, fever, and abdominal cramps in humans, with some cases becoming life-threatening if the infection spreads to the bloodstream. About 1.2 million cases of infection with nontyphoidal *Salmonella* occur annually, causing about 23,000 hospitalizations and

450 deaths. Because *Salmonella* infection is common, the growth of antibiotic-resistant strains of this class of bacteria is of particular concern. About 8 percent of cases of infection with nontyphoidal *Salmonella* show resistance to at least one of the drugs normally used to treat *Salmonella* infections, with 5 percent resistant to at least five classes of antibiotics. Although the number of deaths caused by *Salmonella* infection is relatively low, infection with drug-resistant *Salmonella* tends to result in less effective treatment, resulting in increased probability of hospitalization for patients and increased costs to the healthcare system.

Infections with *Salmonella serotype typhi* (the type of salmonella that causes typhoid fever) cause about 5,700 cases of illness annually in the United States, resulting in 620 hospitalizations, but no more than 5 deaths. Although typhoid fever is a relatively rare disease in the United States, with most cases occurring in people who contracted it while in other countries, it is a serious health threat globally, with about 21.7 million cases occurring annually around the world. Antibiotics have sharply reduced the death toll for this disease (before the use of antibiotics, 10 to 20 percent of people with typhoid fever died from it), but the growth of drug-resistant strains of *S. serotype typhi* raises the possibility that death rates will increase again as current treatments become ineffective. In the United States, about two-thirds of cases of infection with *S. serotype typhi* show at least partial resistance to ciprofloxacin, but they can be treated effectively with ceftriaxone or azithromycin. However, resistance to the latter two drugs has been observed in other parts of the world, and this type of drug resistance also could occur in the United States. In addition, drug-resistant strains of this disease could be brought to the United States by travelers who were infected with it in other countries.

Shigella is a type of bacteria that can cause severe diarrhea, fever, and abdominal pain, and also can cause serious complications, such as reactive arthritis. About 500,000 *Shigella* infections occur annually in the United States, resulting in 5,500 hospitalizations and 40 deaths. *Shigella* strains common in the United States are sufficiently resistant to drugs formerly used as first-line treatments, such as ampicillin, that other drugs such as ciprofloxacin and azithromycin are now commonly used instead. However, strains resistant to these drugs are also emerging, with 2 percent of infections resistant to ciprofloxacin and 3 percent to azithromycin. While *Shigella* infection rarely results in death in the United States, infection with drug-resistant strains increase healthcare costs and may require patients to undergo treatment for a longer period of time.

MRSA is a type of *Staphylococcus* bacteria (staph) that is resistant to methicillin and related antibiotics formerly effective against it. It can cause a wide variety of illnesses, including pneumonia, skin and wound infections, and bloodstream infections. The most severe infections typically occur during care in hospitals or other healthcare settings (e.g., long-term-care homes), while infections in the community are more likely to result in less serious consequences, such as boils. MRSA is a common cause of healthcare-related infection, with the CDC estimating that over 80,000 severe MRSA infections and over 11,000 deaths occurred in the United States in 2011. MRSA infection has declined in recent years, from about 110,000 cases in 2005 to about 80,000 in 2011, but still remains a threat.

S. pneumoniae is a major cause of ear and sinus infections and bloodstream infections in the United States, and it is also the leading cause of bacterial pneumonia and meningitis. About 4 million cases and 22,000 deaths occur annually in the United States due to infection with this pathogen. About 30 percent of infections with S. pneumoniae are caused by strains resistant to one or more types of antibiotics, including the penicillin and erythromycin groups. This is of particular concern because infection with S. pneumoniae is so common: for instance, it is a common cause of ear infections (otitis media) in children, with about 1.5 million cases annually requiring treatment with antibiotics. The most serious disease associated with S. pneumoniae is pneumonia, with about 160,000 children and 600,000 adults treated annually for this disease. The emergence of drug-resistant strains of S. pneumoniae is associated with increased treatment length and costs, and the CDC estimates that the excess costs due to drug-resistant pneumococcal pneumonia alone amounts to about $96 million per year.

TB is caused by infection with the bacteria *Mycobacterium tuberculosis*, which can occur in many parts of the body but occurs most commonly in the lungs. While TB remains a leading cause of death and disability worldwide, effective treatment with antibiotics has greatly reduced its threat to human health in the United States. However, the emergence of drug-resistant strains of TB has raised the possibility that this disease may become a serious health threat in the United States once again. In 2011, 10,528 cases of TB were reported in the United States, of which 9.9 percent showed resistance to at least one antibiotic; the most common type of resistance was to the first-line treatment drug isoniazid. Drug-resistant TB is more expensive to treat and may require a longer treatment period, and the emergence of strains of TB resistant to multiple drugs formerly effective against it means that some cases may simply become untreatable.

Concerning Threats

Three pathogens have been classified as concerning threats: vancomycin-resistant *S. aureus* (VRSA), erythromycin-resistant Group A *Streptococcus*, and clindamycin-resistant Group B *Streptococcus*. For these pathogens, the current level of antibiotic resistance is low, there currently exist multiple effective treatments for diseases caused by antimicrobial-resistant strains of these pathogens, or both. However, these pathogens still require monitoring to assess their ongoing level of threat, and they also may require a rapid response to contain potential outbreaks of infection.

S. aureus is a type of staph bacteria commonly found on the skin, but it can cause severe infections in humans if it is allowed to enter the body. Some strains of *S. aureus* have become resistant to multiple types of antibiotics, as noted earlier in this chapter. For these resistant infections, vancomycin is a common treatment. However, infection with VRSA has been identified in the United States, meaning that this treatment option is no longer effective in these cases. VRSA is currently rare, with only 13 cases identified in the United States between 2002 and 2013, and none resulted in death. However, should infection with VRSA become more common, it would pose an extreme health hazard due to the lack of effective treatment options.

Streptococcus is a type of bacteria responsible for many common infections. Infections with streptococcus are classified into eight groups, labeled as Groups A through H; Groups A and B pose the most concern as far as drug resistance is concerned. Group A *Streptococcus* (GAS) is responsible for illnesses such as strep throat (pharyngitis), scarlet fever, rheumatic fever, the skin infection impetigo, and necrotizing fasciitis (also called "flesh-eating disease"). GAS is responsible for millions of infections annually in the United States, including up to 2.6 million cases of strep throat. GAS has developed resistance to tetracycline, clindamycin, and the macrolide class of drugs, which includes erythromycin and azithromycin. In 2011 and 2012, about 12 percent of GAS bacteria analyzed by the CDC were resistant to erythromycin and other macrolides, while 3.4 percent were resistant to clindamycin. Although the current rate of antibiotic-resistant GAS is low (about 1,300 cases, resulting in 160 deaths annually), the widespread nature of GAS infection means that increased drug resistance could affect large numbers of people. Of particular concern is the possibility that GAS could become resistant to penicillins such as amoxicillin, which are currently a first-line treatment for strep infections.

Group B *Streptococcus* (GBS) can cause a number of diseases in humans, including pneumonia, meningitis, skin infections, and bloodstream infections (sepsis), and it is the leading cause of bacterial infections in newborns. About 27,000 cases of disease caused by severe GBS were recorded in the United States in 2011, causing 1,575 deaths; of those cases, about 7,600 illnesses and 440 deaths were attributable to drug-resistant GBS. The most common types of drug resistance for GBS are resistance to erythromycin (49 percent of drug-resistant GBS samples), which means that the bacteria is also resistant to azithromycin; and resistance to clindamycin (28 percent of drug-resistant GBS samples). Both types of resistance have been increasing since 2000. In addition, a small number of GBS samples are also resistant to vancomycin, an antibiotic currently used as a treatment of last resort. If the proportion of vancomycin-resistant GBS increases, this could create a severe public health problem, as there might be infections for which none of the available antibiotics are effective.

CHAPTER 4

Specific Diseases

Many specific microbes have become resistant to various types of antibiotics. The extent of this problem, both globally and in the United States, was described in Chapter 3. This chapter focuses on several specific diseases that are important threats to human health and for which drug-resistant strains of the causal pathogen are a public health concern.

TUBERCULOSIS

Tuberculosis (TB) is caused by *Mycobacterium tuberculosis*, a type of bacteria that usually attacks the lungs but also can attack other parts of the body, including the spine and brain. TB infection can be fatal, and prior to the introduction of antibiotics effective in treating it, TB patients often died. For this reason, the emergence of strains of TB that are resistant to current antibiotic therapies is a particular cause for concern.

TB is spread through the air when a person infected with the bacteria releases it by coughing, sneezing, or speaking. Someone nearby then may inhale the air containing the bacteria and become infected. Not everyone who is infected with TB gets sick from it, and a positive test for the TB bacteria does not mean that the individual is sick. Some people who test positive have a latent infection, meaning that they have the bacteria in their body but their immune system has been able to keep the bacteria from reproducing sufficiently to make them sick. Someone with a latent infection cannot infect other people with TB; however, if an infected person's immune system cannot fight off the bacteria, the disease will become active, so the person will become sick and then will be capable of spreading the disease to other people.

Some people become ill soon after infection with the TB bacteria, while others may have the bacteria in their system for years, only becoming ill at a much later date (if at all). Risk factors for developing TB after being infected with the TB bacteria include HIV infection, previous recent TB infection (within six months), other health problems like diabetes, abuse of alcohol or illegal drugs, and previous TB infection that was not treated appropriately and hence not entirely cured. Individuals with latent TB infection may be treated with medicine to reduce the probability that they will develop active TB in the future.

Effective treatment of TB requires that the patient follow a course of treatment, usually involving several drugs and requiring 6 to 12 months of treatment. Although patients may feel better early in the treatment course, it is important for them to stay on their prescribed regimen for the entire course of treatment in order to kill the bacteria completely and avoid encouraging the growth of drug-resistant species of TB. The need for a patient to take medication consistently and over a long period of time led to the development of new ways of supervising treatment, including directly observed therapy (DOT), in which the patient takes all required medications in the presence of a nurse or other healthcare worker.

Disease Burden of TB

TB is a relatively rare disease in the United States, with 9,582 cases reported in 2013 (3.0 cases per 100,000 people). Death from TB in the United States is also rare, with 555 deaths from TB in 2013 (the most recent year for which data is available). The TB rate has declined consistently in the United States since 1992, with fewer cases each year, and the death rate from TB also has declined, with a 69 percent decrease from 1992 to 2013. TB is much more common among foreign-born persons, with a case rate of 15.6 cases per 100,000 persons, than among U.S.-born persons (1.2 cases per 100,000). The rate of TB also differs by race and ethnicity, with Asians the most likely to have the disease (18.7 cases per 100,000), followed by native Hawaiians and Pacific Islanders (11.3 cases per 100,000), American Indians and Alaska Natives (5.4 cases per 100,000), Blacks and African Americans (5.4 cases per 100,000), Hispanics and Latinos of any race (5.0 cases per 100,000), and Whites (0.7 cases per 100,000).

Worldwide, TB presents a serious threat to health in many countries, and it is the second-most-deadly infectious disease, after HIV/AIDS. The World Health Organization (WHO) estimates that about one-third of the world's population has latent TB, with about a 10 percent chance of developing active TB at some point in their lives. In 2013, an estimated 9 million people, including 550,000 children aged 0–14 years, contracted TB, and 1.5 million people died of it, including 80,000 HIV-negative children. Most TB cases and deaths occur in low- and middle-income countries, with the greatest number of new cases in 2013 coming from countries in Southeast Asia and the Western Pacific regions.

Due to their weakened immune system, people infected with HIV have a much higher risk (by 28 to 31 times) of developing active TB than are people without HIV infection. About one-quarter of all deaths to people infected with HIV are due to TB. In 2013, HIV-positive people developed an estimated 1.1 million new cases of TB, with the highest proportion (78 percent) of them living in Africa.

Although TB remains a major cause of disease and death in many countries, improved diagnosis and treatment services have resulted in a substantial reduction in the death rate, which fell 45 percent between 1990 and 2013. The WHO estimates that 37 million lives were saved between 2000 and 2013 alone, thanks to diagnosis and treatment of TB.

Drug-Resistant TB

The growth of drug-resistant strains of TB threatens current efforts to fight this disease. As early as the 1940s, when the first clinical trials were being conducted for antibiotic TB treatments, strains of TB resistant to streptomycin were detected in many patients. In every country surveyed by the WHO, strains of TB that have become resistant to at least one drug formerly used to treat the disease have been identified. For this reason, the illness is normally treated with combinations of drugs, with a common regimen today involving rifampicin, isoniazid, ethambutol, and pyrazinamide. Multidrug-resistant TB (MDR-TB), which does not respond to either isoniazid or rifampicin, two common first-line drugs used to treat TB, has been identified in many countries. Although MDR-TB can be treated by other, second-line drugs, those drugs are more expensive, require longer periods of treatment, are less likely to be available, and sometimes evoke serious adverse reactions in patients. In 2013, 480,000 new cases of MDR-TB were identified globally, with over half in just three countries: China, India, and Russia. MDR-TB is relatively rare in the United States, with only 86 cases in 2012 and 95 in 2013. Most cases of MDR-TB (89.5 percent in 2013) in the United States occur in foreign-born persons.

Some strains of TB have become resistant not only to the first-line drugs isoniazid and rifampicin, but also to commonly used second-line drugs. These strains are called *extensively drug-resistant TB (XDR-TB)*. XDR-TB is relatively rare globally, accounting for about 43,200 new cases in 2013.

It is quite uncommon in the United States, with only 63 cases reported between 1993 and 2011. However, XDR-TB is a matter of public health concern because it is difficult to treat effectively with currently existing drugs, and due to air travel, patients infected with XDR-TB may easily carry the infection from one country to another in a different part of the world. By 2013, at least one case of XDR-TB had been reported in 92 countries.

Should MDR-TB or XDR-TB become widespread, medical resources would be strained, and the previous progress made in fighting TB could be reversed. While most cases of susceptible TB (i.e., strains that have not developed drug resistance) can be cured through proper treatment, less than half (48 percent) of persons infected with MDR-TB who began treatment in 2010 were cured at the completion of their course of treatment, and treatment success was even less common for cases of XDR-TB.

GONORRHEA

Gonorrhea is a sexually transmitted disease caused by infection with the bacteria *Neisseria gonorrhoeae.* Gonorrhea is spread primarily through sexual intercourse and oral sex, and it also may be transmitted from mother to child during birth. While gonorrhea may result in infertility for both men and women, other clinical manifestations of gonorrhea differ between the genders. For men, symptoms include a discharge from the urethra, epididymitis (inflammation of the epididymis, a coiled, sperm-carrying tube behind the testicles), and orchitis (inflammation of the testicles). For women, symptoms include cervicitis (inflammation of the cervix, the end of the uterus opening into the vagina), endometritis (inflammation of the lining of the uterus), salpingitis (inflammation of the fallopian tubes), pelvic inflammatory disease (PID), perihepatitis (inflammation of the coating of the liver), and premature rupture of membranes during pregnancy. An estimated 40 percent of women with gonorrhea will develop PID, and about one in four of those with PID will become infertile. Babies infected with gonorrhea may develop conjunctivitis, corneal scarring, and blindness.

The primary methods to prevent infection with gonorrhea are quick and effective treatment of infected individuals and the use of barrier methods, such as condoms, to prevent person-to-person transmission. However, many people infected with gonorrhea are asymptomatic, making diagnosis and treatment difficult: the WHO estimates that 30 to 80 percent of women and 5 percent of men with genital gonorrhea have no symptoms. The fact that so many cases are asymptomatic also makes it difficult to determine how many people contract gonorrhea in a given year, since many infected people may not be aware of their infection and may not seek medical treatment.

Disease Burden of Gonorrhea

Gonorrhea is a notifiable disease in the United States, meaning that cases of gonorrhea must be reported to health authorities. In other countries, this is not necessarily the case, making it difficult to determine how many people are infected with the disease. In addition, because gonorrhea frequently produces no symptoms, as stated previously, many people infected with it may not be aware of that fact and may not seek medical treatment. For these reasons, while information about reported cases of the disease may exist, any information about incidence and prevalence (including unreported and reported cases) can only be estimates.

In the United States, according to the Centers for Disease Control and Prevention (CDC), the rate of reported cases in 2014 was 110.7 per 100,000 population (350,062 total cases)—a small decrease from 2013 (105.3/100,000), but a substantial increase from 2009 (98.1/100,000). In 2014, the rate of reported cases was higher for men (120.1/100,000) than for women (101.3/100,000), although this difference could be partly because women are more likely to experience no symptoms following infection, so they do not report the disease or seek treatment. The case rate was highest among young adults, with 340.7 cases per 100,000 in the 15–19 age group, 495.9/100,000 in the 20–24 age group, and 287.8/100,000 in the 25–29 age group. Case rates generally decline with age: for the 30–34 age group, the case rate was 160.2/100,000; for 25–29, it was 92.0/100,000, for 40–44, it was 45.7/100,000; for ages 45–54, it was 31.6/100,000; for ages 55–62, it was 9.7/100,000, and for those age 65 and older, it was 1.8/100,000.

The WHO estimates that in 2008, 106.1 million new cases of gonorrhea were contracted, a 21 percent increase from the 2005 estimate of 87.7 million. In addition, the WHO estimates that at any moment during that year, 36.4 million people were infected with gonorrhea (because the disease is still largely treatable, those who sought medical care did not have the disease for the entire year). The incidence (of new cases) in 2008 varied by WHO region (highest in the African region, and lowest in the European and Eastern Mediterranean regions), and also by gender (generally higher for men). In the African region, the incidence of gonorrhea was 49.7 cases per 1,000 people for women, and 60.3 per 1,000 for men. In the Americas, the incidence was 18.5/1,000 for women and 27.6 for men. In Southeast Asia, the incidence was 16.2/1,000 for women and 37.0/1,000 for men. In Europe, the incidence was 8.3/1,000 for women and 7.0/1,000 for men. In the Eastern Mediterranean region, the incidence was 8.1/1,000 for women and 11.6/1,000 for men. In the Western Pacific region, the incidence was 34.9/1,000 for women and 49.9/1,000 for men.

Drug-Resistant Gonorrhea

In the past, a number of drugs have been used successfully to treat gonorrhea, including penicillin, sulfonilamides, tetracyclines, and fluoroquinolones (including ciproflaxacin). In the 1990s, the primary drugs used to treat gonorrhea were ciprofloxacin and two drugs in the cephalosporin class, ceftriaxone and cefixime. However, strains of *N. gonorrhoeae* resistant to ciprofloxacin were detected in the United States beginning in the late 1990s, and by 2006, ciprofloxacin had been reported in all regions of the country. In 2007, the CDC no longer recommended the use of fluoroquinolones, including ciprofloxacin, to treat gonorrhea, leaving cefiximim and ceftriaxone as the only remaining effective treatments.

To slow the development of cephalosporin-resistant gonorrhea, the CDC in 2010 began recommending the use of two drugs to treat gonorrhea, as well as increasing the recommended dose of ceftriaxone to 250 mg. As of 2015, the recommended treatment for gonorrhea is dual therapy with oral azithromycin and injectable ceftriaxone. While no treatment failures for gonorrhea have been reported in the United States as of 2016, should *N. gonorrhoeae* develop resistance to the cephalosporins, there will be no effective treatment for gonorrhea among existing drugs.

Globally, strains of *N. gonorrhoeae* resistant to quinolones are also widespread, as is the emergence of strains with decreasing susceptibility to third-generation cephalosporins. As of 2016, the WHO recommends that treatment for genital gonorrhea be based on information about local resistance patterns if possible. Recommended single therapy (using only one drug), based on local resistance data, is either ceftriaxone (250 mg injected), cefime (400 mg orally), or spectinomycin (2 g injected). If local resistance data is not available, the WHO recommends dual therapy with either injectable ceftriaxone plus oral azithromycin, or oral cefixime plus oral azithromycin. For neonates (newborns), the WHO recommends ocular prophylaxis with tetracycline hydrochloride ointment, erythromycin ointment, water-based povidone iodine solution, silver nitrate solution, or chloramphenicol ointment.

MALARIA

Malaria is caused by infection with the *Plasmodium* parasite, which is transmitted through the bite of the female of certain species of the *Anopheles* mosquito. Most human species of malaria are caused by one of four species of *Plasmodium*: *Plasmodium falciparum*, *Plasmodium vivax*, *Plasmodium malariae*, and *Plasmodium oviale*. A fifth species, *Plasmodium knowlesi*, which is primarily associated with malaria in monkeys, also has caused a few human cases of malaria. Infection with *P. falciparum* or *P. vivax* is most common, and infection with *P. falciparum* is associated with the highest rates of severe illness and death from malaria. Once a person is infected with the *Plasmodium* parasite, it travels through the individual's bloodstream to the liver, where it multiplies. The parasite then attacks red blood cells, and the resulting disease is characterized by high fevers, chills, and flulike symptoms.

Malaria can be treated with various drug therapies, but it can be fatal if not treated. Providing prompt and effective treatment is also important because reducing the number of cases of malaria in a population is one key to malaria control. This is because mosquitoes can contract the parasite by biting an infected human, and then transmit it to other humans by biting them, so more infected people mean more opportunities for mosquitoes to contract the disease and spread it. Should the drugs currently used to treat malaria become ineffective, the result could be widespread disease and death in areas where malaria is endemic (i.e., where it regularly occurs).

Malaria presently is not a major health threat in the United States, with about 1,500 cases reported each year, mostly from travelers or immigrants who have been in countries where malaria is common, particularly those in South Asia and sub-Saharan Africa. However, in parts of the world, malaria remains a serious health threat. For instance, in 2015, the WHO estimated that 3.2 billion people (about half of the world's population) are at risk of contracting malaria. The WHO estimated that in 2015, there were about 214 million malaria cases globally, and about 438,000 deaths from malaria. Most (89 percent) cases and most (91 percent) malaria deaths were in sub-Saharan Africa, with children and pregnant women being at greatest risk. The direct cost of malaria, including the costs of treating the illness and burying the dead, have been estimated to be at least $12 billion annually; the cost to economic growth (e.g., through lost productivity) is more difficult to calculate, but it is assumed to be many times higher.

Drug-Resistant Malaria

Drug resistance in malaria is somewhat complicated to evaluate because it cannot be identified through a simple lab test. Instead, it is identified through the lack of effectiveness of treatment: If the *Plasmodium* parasite survives and multiplies despite the administration of drugs formerly successful in treating malaria in the doses usually administered, that is taken as evidence of resistance. However, evaluating drug resistance is also complicated by the fact that the pharmacokinetic properties (i.e., the way that drugs are absorbed, distributed, metabolized, and excreted by an individual) of antimalarial drugs can vary widely from one person to another, making treatment more complicated. For this reason, the concentration of the drug in an individual's blood or plasma must be monitored to be sure that it is at a therapeutic level, because administering a standard dose of the drug may have different results for different people.

Strains of malaria resistant to the drugs commonly used to treat the disease were first identified in the 1970s, when strains of *P. falciparum* resistant to chloroquine and pyrimethamine were detected in Southeast Asia. Strains of malaria resistant to those drugs that were commonly used to treat the disease at the time then spread to Africa. In the 1980s, strains of *P. falciparum* resistant to mefloquine were detected in Cambodia and Thailand only a few years after the introduction of that drug to treat malaria. In the 1990s, strains of *P. falciparum* that were resistant to amodiaquine and sulfadoxine-pyrimethamine (a combination drug sold under the brand name Fansidar) were discovered.

Because of the demonstrated ability of the *Plasmodium* parasite to develop resistance quickly, malaria today is generally treated with a combination of drugs. The principle of combination therapy, which is also used to treat illnesses such as HIV, TB, and leprosy, is that the use of two or more drugs with different modes of action will slow the development of drug-resistant organisms. One drug commonly used to treat malaria is artemisinin, a substance isolated from the sweet wormwood (*Artemisia annua*) plan. Artemisinin and its derivatives act quickly to kill the *Plasmodium* parasites, but they are also rapidly eliminated from the body, while the person still may be infected with parasites that can then continue to replicate and thus cause further illness. For this reason, artemisinin is generally combined with another drug that acts more slowly but remains in the body longer, such as lumefantrine, mefloquine, or piperaquine, so that the parasites not killed by the artemesinin will be killed by the slower-acting drug.

Artemisinin-based combination therapy (ACT) has become a mainstay of antimalarial treatment, with 392 million ACT treatment courses delivered in 2013 (by comparison, only 11 million ACT treatment courses were delivered in 2005). Five different courses of ACT are currently available. However, in some countries, treatment with artemisinin alone (artemisinin-based monotherapy) is still used, a practice that encourages the development of artemisinin-resistant *Plasmodium* parasites.

Because ACT is the most common and antimalarial treatment today, the development of artemisinin-resistant strains of *Plasmodium* is a major public health concern. While there are treatments other than artemisinin available for malaria, none are as effective, or are tolerated as well by patients, as ACT. As of February 2015, artemisinin resistance has been located in only one geographic area: the Greater Mekong subregion, which includes parts of five countries: Cambodia. Laos, Myanmar (Burma), Thailand, and Vietnam. Even in this region, however, most patients treated for malaria still recover from the disease after being treated with ACT. However, a strain of *P. falciparum* resistant to almost all antimalarial medicines has been discovered in an area on the border between Cambodia and Thailand. Should this strain spread to other parts of the world, or should other strains resistant to artemisinin emerge, the public health consequences could be severe.

HIV

HIV impairs and destroys the cells of the immune system, leaving an infected person vulnerable to many infections that can be resisted by a person with a normal immune system. In most people, the virus progresses if untreated, destroying the infected person's immune system and leading to the development of AIDS. HIV is spread through the exchange of bodily fluids, which may occur during various activities, including sexual relations, childbirth, breastfeeding, needle sharing, and some medical procedures.

So far as we know, HIV infection in humans is a relatively new phenomenon, and awareness of AIDS is also relatively recent. The first published report of AIDS occurred in 1981, when several articles described young men in the United States diagnosed with diseases generally unknown among young people with healthy immune systems, including *Pneumocystis carinii* pneumonia (PCP) and Kaposi's sarcoma, a type of skin cancer. Because these early cases occurred in gay men, the condition was initially labeled "gay-related immune deficiency (GRID)." As cases were identified in people other than gay men, the name of the condition was changed to AIDS. The states of being infected with HIV and having AIDS are often grouped together in statistical reporting, with both conditions referred to jointly as *HIV/AIDS*.

Although there is currently no cure for AIDS, the development of antiretroviral therapy (ART) to treat HIV infection in the 1990s was a major breakthrough. The availability of treatment with ART changed HIV infection and AIDS from a likely death sentence to a chronic disease. Treatment with ART also helps contain the spread of HIV by making treated people less likely to pass the disease on to others. ART drugs fight HIV by preventing the virus from replicating in an infected person's body, thus reducing the viral load (the amount of virus present in the person's body). Five main classes of antiretrovirals are used to treat HIV infection and AIDS: nucleoside/nucleotide reverse transcriptase inhibitors (NRTIs), nonnucleoside reverse transcriptase inhibitors (NNRTIs), protease inhibitors (PIs), entry/fusion inhibitors, and integrase inhibitors. ART is usually delivered through combination therapy involving at least three antiretroviral drugs, and it is used both to treat people infected with HIV (including those suffering from AIDS) and as a preventative treatment, particularly for pregnant women.

Number of Cases

Globally, about 35 million people are currently living with HIV/AIDS, including 3.2 million children younger than 15, and an additional 2.1 million people became newly infected in 2013, including 240,000 children. AIDS is the world's deadliest infectious disease, with 1.5 million deaths worldwide from AIDS-related causes in 2013. Most people living with HIV/AIDS live in low- or middle-income countries, and 71 percent of people living with HIV/AIDS are in sub-Saharan Africa.

In the United States, over 1.2 million people are living with HIV/AIDS. About 50,000 new cases of HIV infection are identified each year (44,073 in 2014), but because infected people are living longer due to better treatments, the total number of people living with HIV/AIDS increases each year. In 2013, 6,995 people died from HIV and AIDS in the United States. The risk of HIV/AIDS is not spread evenly across the population, with gay and bisexual men, injection drug users, African Americans, and Hispanics/Latinos having an elevated risk of being affected by HIV/AIDS.

Drug Resistance

Mutation is common in HIV because the virus replicates rapidly. While the development of drug resistance is expected in all microbes, due to the normal process of evolution, the rapid rate of mutation in HIV means that it is particularly apt at developing strains resistant to drugs used to treat HIV. Two types of drug resistance have been identified for HIV: transmitted HIV drug resistance and acquired HIV drug resistance. Transmitted HIV drug resistance occurs when an individual is infected with a strain of HIV that has already become drug resistant. Acquired HIV drug resistance occurs when drug resistance occurs during treatment due to resistant, mutated strains of HIV being selected for survival during ART treatment.

Surveys conducted by WHO have found increasing levels of resistance to one of the classes of drugs used to treat HIV/AIDS, NNRTIs, among HIV-infected patients who have not yet begun treatment with ART. NNRTI resistance was highest in Africa (at 3.4 percent of cases). The overall rate of drug resistance (to any antiretroviral drug) in low- and middle-income countries among patients beginning ART was estimated at 4.8 percent in 2010. ART treatment is still effective for about 90 percent of people with HIV/AIDS, by the standard that their viral load was lowered 12 months after beginning treatment. However, among the 10 percent for whom treatment was not successful, 72 percent have resistance to at least one anti-retroviral drug, usually of the NRTI or NNRTI class.

The development of effective treatments for AIDS is one of the most important medical breakthroughs of the late 20th and early 21st centuries. However, this success has been due in large part to increased use of ART, and this has created the conditions for increased resistance to the drugs used in ART. Some resistance to classes of ART drugs has already been identified, and the spread of drug-resistant strains of HIV could threaten the success currently seen in limiting the effects of HIV/AIDS.

If the drugs currently used to treat HIV/AIDS become ineffective, not only will the individuals already infected suffer from the lack of effective treatments to lower their viral load and thus prevent the progression to AIDS, but they will also remain more likely to infect others and thus increase the rate of HIV infection. A second concern is that because HIV/AIDS cannot be cured, patients must continue taking medications for the rest of their lives to suppress the virus. If the medications become ineffective, the patients are likely to suffer relapses and perhaps progress to full-blown AIDS. Finally, alternative treatments of AIDS are limited and considerably more expensive than currently effective treatments, placing a greater strain on national health budgets and possibly limiting the availability of effective treatments in some parts of the world if it becomes necessary to switch to these more expensive treatments.

INFLUENZA

Influenza (flu) is a disease caused by a virus that most commonly affects the nose, throat, and bronchi, and may attack the lungs as well. Flu is a common disease, with most cases occurring during the winter season (December through March in the northern hemisphere, April through September in the southern hemisphere). The severity of an individual case of the flu can range from relatively mild to extremely serious, and while most cases resolve without medical intervention, severe cases of the flu can be fatal. Typical symptoms of the flu include a sore throat, cough, runny nose, body aches, and headache, and children and infants also may exhibit vomiting and diarrhea.

Flu usually spreads quickly through a population, in part because an infected person can transmit the disease to others during the incubation period, when the infected person has no symptoms of the disease. The attack rate (the proportion of exposed individuals who become ill) is usually in the range of 10 to 30 percent annually, with higher attack rates for children than for adults. Flu is transmitted by respiratory secretions emitted from coughing or sneezing, or by touching the nose or mouth. Frequently, it is spread through secondary contact, in which the infected person has flu virus on the hands, touches a surface, and then an uninfected person touches the same surface and then touches the nose or eyes, thus becoming infected. In addition, some types of flu can be spread from animals to humans, such as some types of avian (bird) flu.

The annual outbreaks of flu are usually caused by one of two types of the virus, Type A or Type B, and the flu vaccine is engineered to offer protection against these types of flu. The type A virus is further divided into subtypes, according to two proteins found on the surface of the virus: hemagglutinin (H) and neuraminidase (N). For instance, two types of avian flu that can infect humans are both Type A, but with different subtypes, classified as A(H5N1) and A(H7N9). In total, 17 H subtypes and 10 N subtypes of the flu are currently known.

Number of Cases

In a typical year, about 3 to 5 million cases of serious illness each year are caused by the flu virus, and 250,000 to 500,000 people die from it. The risk of death from the flu is greatest for children under the age of 2, people over the age of 65, pregnant women, and people with certain chronic diseases or weakened immune systems. However, sometimes a strain of the flu can be much deadlier: for instance, an estimated 50 million people died during the 1918–1919 Spanish flu pandemic (a widespread or worldwide outbreak of disease). In the United States, about 200,000 people are hospitalized annually with severe cases of the flu, and about 36,000 die from it.

Vaccines and Treatment

The primary public health method to control flu outbreaks, besides modifying behavior (i.e., staying home while ill, covering your mouth when you cough, and avoiding touching your eyes or nose), is the widespread administration of the flu vaccine. Preparing the flu vaccine is a tricky process because the type of flu that are most common change from year to year, and the process of creating the vaccine begins about six months before the annual flu season. The vaccine is most effective when well matched with the specific strains of flu most active in a given year, a fact that cannot be known when production of the vaccine begins. Therefore, the scientists involved in creating the vaccine each year must try to predict which specific types and subtypes will be most problematic in the upcoming flu season and create a vaccine effective against those subtypes. In addition, flu viruses are constantly evolving, so even within a subtype, a virus that is active in a given year may be substantially different from previous versions of the same subtype.

In 2014, the WHO recommended an annual flu vaccination for pregnant women, healthcare workers, people with chronic medical conditions, people over the age of 65, and children aged 6 months to 5 years. In some countries, such as the United States, recommendations for annual flu vaccination extend to even more people. For instance, the CDC recommends an annual flu vaccination for everyone living in the United States aged 6 months and older except for a few groups of people, including those with allergies to eggs or other ingredients used in making the vaccine.

For people who already have the flu, a few treatments are available in some countries. All involve the administration of antiviral drugs (drugs that are effective against viruses), preferably within 48 hours of the onset of flu symptoms. These drugs can reduce the duration of illness by one to two days on average and lessen the probability that the infected person will develop a secondary bacterial infection. In addition, antiviral drugs can lessen the risk of flu infection if taken prophylactically.

Two classes of antiviral drugs are currently used to treat the flu: adamantanes (including amantadine and rimantadine) and influenza N inhibitors (including oseltamivir, zanamivir, peramivir, and laninamivir). However, adamantine resistance developed rapidly in the first decade of the 21st century and became fixed in the A(H3N2) virus during the 2004–2005 flu season. In 2009, the A(H1N1) virus also acquired resistance to adamantine. Because adamantine resistance developed so rapidly and is now widespread around the world, these drugs are not currently recommended by WHO for use against seasonal influenza viruses.

Oseltamivir and zanamivir, both neuraminidase inhibitors developed in the 1990s, are widely used and effective against both Type A and Type B influenza viruses. Oseltamivir is the treatment of choice in many countries that have stockpiled antiviral drugs for pandemic preparedness, so the development of resistant strains of flu would present a problem to public health efforts. Resistance varies depending on the strain of the flu virus, but two strains already show some resistance to oseltamivir. In particular, the emergence of A(H1N1) resistance to oseltamivir in 2007–2008 suggests that the flu virus can be expected to develop resistance to this class of drugs as well. Another strain of flu, A(H1N1), currently has low resistance to oseltamivir (1 to 3 percent), but any resistance is worrying. If more strains develop resistance to neuraminidase inhibitors, it would severely limit efforts to treat patients who have contracted the flu.

CHAPTER 5

Measures to Combat Drug Resistance

Drug resistance is an increasing threat to human health, but there are many measures available to help reduce and contain the growth of drug-resistant organisms. One major approach is to rationalize the use of antibiotics in human medicine by educating physicians, dispensers, and patients as to the appropriate use of these drugs. Other measures centering on the healthcare system include using appropriate infection control procedures, promoting vaccination programs, and improving surveillance and reporting programs. Developing new antibiotics and improved diagnostic tests also plays a key role in combating antibiotic resistance, as does implementing appropriate measures to limit the spread of disease through travel.

NATIONAL AND INTERNATIONAL STANDARDS OF PRESCRIBING PRACTICE

Antibiotics have saved millions of lives since their introduction in the 1940s, and the development of effective antibiotic treatments can rightfully be regarded as one of the greatest accomplishments of modern medical practice. However, disease-causing bacteria also have displayed a great ability to become resistant to the drugs used against them, and greater use of antibiotics is associated with quicker development of resistance. For this reason, preventing the overuse of antibiotics is a key strategy in helping limit or slow the growth of antibiotic resistance.

Various studies have found that physicians frequently prescribe antibiotics when they are not needed. Some studies have found that the incorrect use of antibiotics accounts for as much as 50 percent of all antibiotic prescriptions if other mistakes, such as prescribing the wrong dose, are included in the tally. While there may be no adverse consequences for each individual patient to taking an antibiotic when it is not needed, from a public health point of view, this is a harmful practice because it encourages the growth of antibiotic-resistant bacteria. The number of antibiotics currently effective against particular types of infections is limited, and each time that a resistant strain emerges, one less tool is available to treat diseases caused by that strain of bacteria.

While it is unlikely that any physician would deliberately misuse antibiotics, wide variations in the number of antibiotics used, relative to the population size, in different U.S. states and different countries, suggest that in at least some cases, the differences may be due to the writing of unnecessary antibiotic prescriptions. For instance, in the United States in 2010, the number of antibiotic prescriptions per person issued ranged from 529 to 1,237 per 1,000 persons. States with the lowest usage included California, Oregon, Washington, Colorado, Vermont, and New Hampshire, while states with the highest usage included North Dakota, Indiana, West Virginia, Kentucky, Tennessee, Arkansas, Louisiana, Mississippi, and Alabama.

While not all the states in either the high or the low group are contiguous (share borders), these statistics do reveal a pattern of antibiotic use being comparatively lower on the West Coast and higher in the Southern states. Possibly these observed differences are due to cultural differences, such as different patient expectations or different medical practices, rather than due to different rates of diseases for which antibiotics are an appropriate treatment.

Antibiotic use can vary widely across different countries as well. For instance, a 2012 surveillance report by the European Centre for Disease Prevention and Control (ECDC) found wide variation in antibiotic use across 30 European countries. Antibiotic use was measured in defined daily doses (DDD), defined as the average maintenance dose per day for adults per 1,000 population.

Across all 30 countries, the average antibiotic use in the community (as opposed to in hospital care) was 21.5 DDD per 1,000 inhabitants. However, use in specific countries varied almost threefold, from 31.9 DDD per 1,000 in Greece to 11.3 DDD per 1,000 in the Netherlands. Although there were no significant trends in antibiotic use when averaged across all the countries, trends were observed in particular countries from 2008 to 2012. Over this time period, five countries (Belgium, Latvia, Norway, Spain, and the United Kingdom) showed a significant increase, and one (Austria) showed a significant decrease. The most commonly used types of antibiotics were penicillins, followed by macrolides and tetracyclines.

Similar ranges were seen in per capita use of antibiotics in the hospital sector. The average use was 2.0 DDD per 1,000 inhabitants, with the greatest use in Finland (2.8 DDD per 1,000) and the lowest in the Netherlands (1.0 DDD per 1,000). The most commonly used antibacterials in the hospital sector were penicillins, followed by other beta-lactam (β-lactam) antibacterials, including quinolones and cephalosporins.

The use of other antimicrobials showed an even wider range. The use of antimycotics and antifungals (both used to combat fungal infections) in the hospital sector varied from 0.03 DDD per 1,000 in Lithuania to 0.2 DDD per 1,000 in Denmark, based on data from 18 countries. The use of antivirals, in both the community and hospital sectors, ranged from 4.4 DDD per 1,000 in Portugal to 0.1 DDD per 1,000 in Malta.

Antibiotic Use in the United States

In the United States, the use of antibiotics is common but has declined over the past several decades. According to data from Centers for Disease Control and Prevention (CDC), published in *Health, United States, 2013*, in the period from 1988 to 1994, 10.1 percent of children and adolescents (under age 18) reported using an antibiotic in the previous 30 days, while in the period from 2007 to 2010, this percentage fell to 6.1 percent. The prescription of antibiotics to treat colds (an incorrect use because colds are caused by a viral infection and thus are not susceptible to antibiotics) also showed a strong decline. In 1995–1996, antibiotics were provided or ordered in 44.7 percent of all physician, outpatient, and emergency visits in which a cold was diagnosed, as compared to 27.1 percent in 2009–2010. For children and adolescents (those under 18 years of age), the percentage of diagnosed colds treated with antibiotics fell from 37.5 percent in 1995–1996 to 21.5 percent in 2009–2010, while for persons 18 years and over, it fell from 58.5 percent in 1995–1996 to 39.5 percent in 2009–2010.

A study of nationally representative data from the Medical Expenditure Panel Survey (MEPS) by Lee et al. (2014) found that antibiotic prescribing in outpatient settings was essentially unchanged from 2000 to 2010. In 2000, 379 prescriptions for antibiotics were issued per 1,000 persons, and 386 prescriptions per 1,000 in 2010 (a statistically insignificant result, meaning that chance could not be ruled out as the cause of the difference in the two figures). However, distinctive patterns were identified among different age groups. For children and adolescents under age 18, a statistically significant decline was observed, with 506 antibiotic prescriptions per 1,000 population in 2000 and 416 per 1,000 in 2010. For adults age 18 to 64, there was no statistically significant change, with 328 antibiotic prescriptions per 1,000 population in 2000 and 354 per 1,000 in 2010. Finally, for adults age 65 and older, antibiotic use increased during this period, with a statistically significant change from 369 antibiotic prescriptions per 1,000 population in 2000 to 480 per 1,000 in 2010.

Lee et al. (2014) also found differing patterns of use depending on the type of antibiotic. The use of broad-spectrum antibiotics increased significantly, from 223 prescriptions per 1,000 population in 2000 to 471 per 1,000 in 2010. Antibiotic prescriptions for acute respiratory tract infections (ARTIs), which include the common cold, sinusitis, laryngitis, pharyngitis, and otitis media, which are often caused by viruses rather than bacteria, declined significantly over the same period, from 175 prescriptions per 1,000 population in 2000 to 102 per 1,000 in 2010.

Antibiotic-Prescribing Reform in the United States

In the United States, the CDC assumes a leadership role in the national fight against the transmission of infections in healthcare settings and agriculture, as well as the promotion of healthcare practices that combat the creation and growth of populations of drug-resistance. Among other things, the CDC has created programs such as the National Healthcare Safety Network (NHSN) to track infections, antibiotic use, and the detection of drug-resistant microbes in healthcare settings; operates a national reference laboratory to detect new and emerging resistance patterns; and conducts surveys to estimate the number of healthcare-related infections occurring in the United States and to study the relationship between antibiotic use and healthcare-related infections.

Another way that the CDC takes part in the fight against antimicrobial resistance is through programs to encourage the appropriate use of antibiotics in healthcare and agricultural settings. One example is the Get Smart program, created in 1995, which is conducted at the national level and targets antibiotic-prescribing practices in inpatient (e.g., hospital) and outpatient (e.g., physician's office) settings, as well as in animal husbandry. The Get Smart program includes Get Smart About Antibiotics Week, an annual event each November, which aims to raise awareness about the dangers of antibiotic resistance and improve prescribing practices. The Get Smart program also funds state-based programs working toward these goals, provides information and resources to improve antibiotic use in healthcare settings, and created the Antibiotic Stewardship Drivers and Change Package, which provides a number of interventions that healthcare facilities can use to improve their use of antibiotics.

Treatment Guidelines for Common Infections

The CDC adult guidelines for antibiotic use include basic information about five common conditions often treated with antibiotics: acute rhinosinusitis (inflammation of the sinuses), acute uncomplicated bronchitis (inflammation of the lining of the bronchial tubes, which carry air to and from the lungs), the common cold and similar infections, pharyngitis (sore throat), and acute uncomplicated cystitis (bladder infection). Although all these conditions are commonly treated by antibiotics, antibiotics are not always helpful (for instance, if the symptoms are caused by a viral infection). The guidelines provide specific recommendations to help physicians differentiate between cases where antibiotics would be helpful and those in which they would not.

For acute rhinosinusitis, the guidelines note that 90 to 98 percent of cases are caused by viral infection, in which case antibiotics are not helpful, and also state that rhinosinusitis is extremely common, with over 30 million diagnoses reported in 2012. Diagnosis of a bacterial infection should be based on the persistence of symptoms over multiple days, such as a fever and purulent discharge (a discharge containing pus) for more than 3 or 4 days, worsening symptoms over 3 or 4 days, or symptoms lasting longer than 10 days. Management of a bacterial infection may include watchful waiting (if the case is uncomplicated and follow-up care is available if needed), the use of amoxicillin or amoxicillin/clavulanate as a first-line therapy, and taking doxycycline or a respiratory fluoroquinolone (levofloxacin or moxifloxacin) with patients allergic to penicillin.

For acute uncomplicated bronchitis, a common diagnosis when a patient visits a physician complaining of a cough, the guidelines recommend focusing first on ruling out pneumonia. Pneumonia is a serious but rare disease among healthy adults and one that generally produces specific symptoms, including a fever, elevated heart and respiratory rate, and abnormal lung conditions. The guidelines note that colored sputum (fluid from the respiratory tract produced by a cough) does not necessarily indicate the presence of a bacterial infection. The guidelines advise addressing bronchitis not caused by pneumonia by treating the symptoms rather than prescribing antibiotics; examples of useful symptomatic treatments include cough suppressants such as dextromethorphan or codeine, antihistamines, decongestants such as phenylephrine, and beta agonists such as albuterol.

The common cold and similar nonspecific upper respiratory tract infections are extremely common (most adults experience two to four colds each year) and can be caused by a number of viruses (over 200 viruses have been identified that can cause the common cold and similar infections).

Antibiotics are not useful against viral infections, and the guidelines recommend that the physician and patient discuss the use of symptomatic therapies such as decongestants (e.g., pseudoephedrine or phenylephrine) and nonsteroidal anti-inflammatory drugs (e.g., aspirin and acetaminophen).

For pharyngitis, the guidelines note that only 5 to 10 percent of cases, those caused by a Group A beta-hemolytic *Streptococcus* (GAS) infection, should be considered for antibiotic treatment, while the rest are caused by viruses and thus should not be treated with antibiotics. GAS infections can be identified through a rapid antigen detection test (RADT); such a test should be administered only to patients who have at least two symptoms included in the Centor criteria, a set of clinical signs and symptoms that includes swelling on the tonsils, tender or swollen cervical lymph nodes, fever over 100.4 degrees Fahrenheit, and absence of a cough. Antibiotic treatment is recommended only for patients with positive RADT results, with amoxicillin and penicillin V potassium (penicillin VK) the first-line drugs of choice. For patients allergic to penicillin, macrolides, clindamycin, cefadroxil, and cephalexin are recommended as alternative treatments.

Cystitis, usually caused by *Escherichia coli*, is the most common cause of infections in women. Recommended first-line treatments are nitrofurantoin, trimethoprim/sulfamethoxazole (TMP/SMX), or fosfomycin, with fluoroquinolones such as ciprofloxacin recommended for cases in which the first-line treatments cannot be used.

For children, the Get Smart program has issued a set of treatment recommendations and guidelines for six common infections: acute rhinosinusitis (inflammation of the sinuses); acute otitis media (AOM), a middle ear infection; pharyngitis (sore throat); the common cold and similar upper respiratory infections (URIs); bronchiolitis (inflammation of the bronchioles, small airways leading to the lung); and urinary tract infections (UTIs).

For acute rhinosinusitis, the guidelines note that most (90 to 98 percent) of the cases are caused by a virus and are thus not responsive to antibiotics. A bacterial diagnosis is recommended only if one or more of the following symptoms are present: persistent daytime cough or nasal discharge without improvement for more than 10 days; worsening symptoms, or severe symptoms such as a fever over 102.2 degrees Fahrenheit; or purulent nasal discharge for three or more days in a row. If a bacterial infection is diagnosed, the recommended first-line treatment is amoxicillin or amoxicillin/clavulanate. Several other treatments are possible for children who are hypersensitive to penicillin, and ceftriaxone can be used to treat children who cannot take oral medication (for instance, due to vomiting).

AOM is the most common childhood disease treated with antibiotics. However, frequently antibiotics are not required to treat AOM, and in 4 to

10 percent of cases, antibiotic treatment of AOM results in adverse effects. The treatment guidelines recommend that AOM be diagnosed only when there is middle ear effusion (presence of fluid) and one of the following: moderate or severe bulging of the tympanic membrane (eardrum), discharge from the middle ear not due to infection in the outer ear (otitis externa), or mild bulging of the eardrum and either otalgia (pain in the ear), begun within the last two days, or intense erythema (reddening) of the eardrum. Mild cases of AOM may be treated by watchful waiting, with shared decision making between the parents and physician, or by administering antibiotics. Amoxicillin is the first-line treatment for AOM, with amoxicillin/clavulanate recommended if the patient has had infections resistant to amoxicillin or has taken amoxicillin in the past 30 days. Other possible treatments include cefdinir, cefuroxime, cefpodocime, or ceftriaxone, which are recommended for children with hypersensitivity to penicillin. The prophylactic use of antibiotics to prevent AOM is not recommended by the guidelines.

The guidelines recommend the use of RADT to identify cases of pharyngitis that may be susceptible to antibiotic treatment, while also noting that false positives are common (occurring in up to 20 percent of cases); in addition, the guidelines note that streptococcal pharyngitis is rare in preschool children. RADT is recommended for children reporting a sore throat plus two or more of the following clinical features: history of fever, swollen and tender anterior cervical lymph nodes, lack of cough, and being younger than 15 years old. The first-line therapy for confirmed cases of bacterial pharyngitis are amoxicillin and penicillin VK, with cephalexin, cefadroxil, clindamycin, clarithromycin, or azithromycin recommended for children with non–Type I penicillin hypersensitivity, and clindamycin, clarithyomycin, or azithromycin recommended for those with immediate Type I penicillin hypersensitivity (i.e., the type of sensitivity that manifests itself within a few hours of administration, as opposed to delayed hypersensitivity, which may not be evident for 24 hours or more following administration).

The common cold and nonspecific URIs can be caused by over 200 viruses and generally resolve within 5 to 7 days (URIs) or around 10 days (colds). Antibiotics are not useful against the common cold or URIs, but a number of over-the-counter (OTC) drugs can be used to relieve symptoms. However, there is no evidence that OTC drugs intended to reduce cough and cold symptoms are effective for children under 6 years, and they can carry risks, so their use should be considered carefully.

Bronchiolitis is the most common infection of the lower respiratory tract in infants and is usually caused by a virus, in which case it should not be treated by antibiotics. The mainstay treatment for bronchiolitis is nasal suctioning (removing secretions through a tube in the nose), with other treatments including albuterol (effective in about 1 in 4 children) and nebulized racemic epinephrine also available.

UTIs are common in children, with about 85 percent caused by *E. coli*. Diagnosis is made by urinalysis, with treatment based on knowledge of local patterns of antimicrobial susceptibility. Possible antibiotics for use in treating UTIs include TMP/SMX, amoxicillin/clavulanate, cefixime, cefpodoxime, cefprozil, and cephalexin.

Reducing the Use of Unprescribed Antibiotics

In the United States and many European countries, antibiotics are available only by prescription. However, in many other countries, they are available over the counter and can be purchased without presentation of a physician's prescription (although they might have to be requested from the pharmacist, as opposed to being on open shelves), a situation that can lead to overuse of antibiotics that fosters the growth of drug-resistant microbes. Even when prescription laws limiting access to antibiotics exist, they are not always enforced, particularly in developing countries, and often antibiotics are available without prescription from a variety of sources, from hospitals and pharmacies to unregulated roadside stands. This is a problem because even physicians can mistake a viral infection (which cannot be helped by antibiotics) from an infection caused by bacteria (in which case appropriate antibiotics may help), so it is not surprising that individuals without medical training may take antibiotics inappropriately when deciding on their own course of treatment themselves.

Haak and Radyowijati (2010) that the use of antibiotics, including unprescribed antibiotics, is not a simple issue. While concern about the growth of drug-resistant organisms has sparked interest in limiting inappropriate microbial use, they find that this concern is often misguided and based on incorrect assumptions. For instance, the use of antibiotics without a prescription is often referred to as "self-medication," but in fact, the decision to use antibiotics byr an individual in a developing country may be influenced by many factors. One is advice garnered from informal care networks, such as friends and family members, rather than formal healthcare institutions. Another source of information may be advice from a pharmacist: for instance, pharmacy personnel in Mexico and the Philippines are known to give medical advice to patients, including advising them to take antibiotics. An individual also may be provided with antibiotics by traditional medical practitioners.

Haak and Radyowijati described an "antimicrobial folk culture" that exists in some developing countries, in which high faith is placed in the use of antimicrobials to manage or cure many medical conditions. While sometimes these beliefs are congruent with accepted medical practice, often they are not: for instance, antimicrobials in Vietnam are often used to treat a variety of ailments, including fever, inflammations, diarrhea, and infections. Often, the reason for using the antibiotic is perceived symptoms rather than certain knowledge of the underlying cause—a fever may have many causes, for instance, and antibiotics may be useful in some cases but not others. Sometimes belief in the efficacy of a particular medicine is based not on the active ingredients, but on seemingly unrelated factors such as the color of the capsule, as was found in a 1998 review article by de Craen and colleagues. Antimicrobials may also be taken prophylactically in the belief that they will prevent conditions such as diarrhea, cough, or fever.

Although inappropriate use of antibiotics may harm the individual taking the drugs as well as endangering public health, it is not useful to place the primary blame on the antibiotic user. That individual may be making what he or she thinks is a rational choice, given the available options: for instance, a physician may not be available, or the person may not be able to pay for a clinic visit, so she or he purchases a medicine that may cure the illness. An important aspect of limiting the use of unprescribed antibiotics, therefore, lies in seeing that all people have access to physician's services when they need them, so they can receive professional advice as to which drugs will help cure their illness. Another aspect of the process of limiting the use of unprescribed antibiotics in countries where they are sold over the counter is public education to help individuals understand how antibiotics work, the types of diseases for which they are and are not effective, and the negative consequences of inappropriate antibiotic use. Finally, any campaign to curb the use of unprescribed antibiotics should be aware of the culture, traditions, and economic conditions of the area where it is implemented.

INFECTION CONTROL

One key tool in combating antibiotic resistance is infection control. Following good infection control procedures is particularly important in healthcare settings because many infections with resistant organisms take place in hospitals and other places where healthcare is delivered. An infection that is contracted in a hospital or other healthcare setting is known as a *healthcare-associated infection (HAI)*. Two similar terms are *nosocomial infection*, referring to an infection contracted in a hospital, and *iatrogenic infection*, referring to an infection caused by medical care. Many HAIs are preventable if hospitals and other healthcare locations implement appropriate infection control measures.

Infection control was the concern of some physicians and other healthcare professions even before the mechanisms of disease transmission were fully understood. For instance, in the 18th century, it was common practice in some hospitals for medical students and physicians to move between dissecting cadavers and treating patients without washing their hands or changing their clothing. Hungarian physician Ignaz Semmelweis was able to drastically lower the rate of puerperal fever (also called *childbed fever*) in the Vienna General Hospital by requiring physicians to wash their hands in a chlorinated lime solution between doing autopsy work and delivering babies—a solution reached before Louis Pasteur developed the germ theory of disease later in the century.

In the mid-19th century, Joseph Lister pioneered the process of antiseptic surgery at the Glasgow Royal Infirmary. Lister was aware of Pasteur's work and believed that surgical infections were not due to "bad air" or miasma, a common belief at the time, but to contamination by the surgeon's hands or surgical tools. Lister applied carbolic acid, a chemical used to treat sewage, to wounds and surgical dressings, and also used it to disinfect surgical instruments and the surgeon's hands, measures that resulted in a substantial reduction in infections contracted during and after surgery.

Improved methods of infection control continue to be developed, and various organizations provide education and monitoring to see that the best available methods are appropriately implemented. Despite these improvements, HAIs have not been eliminated: for instance, the World Health Organization (WHO) estimates that, in high-income countries, 7 percent of patients admitted to a hospital will contract at least one HAI, with individuals in intensive care units (ICUs) at greatest risk (about one in three ICU patients will contract at least one HAI, according to WHO estimates). In low- or middle-income countries, the rate of HAIs is even higher: according to WHO estimates, about 10 percent of those admitted to a hospital in a low- or middle-income country will contract at least one HAI.

Therefore, even in countries with advanced medical care, HAIs remain a concern. Many countries have implemented efforts aimed at reducing and eliminating them, and such efforts can result in substantial reductions. For instance, the CDC tracks the occurrence of HAIs in the United States through the NHSN, which gathers information from over 17,000 hospitals and other healthcare facilities. In 2016, the CDC reported that, in the United States, there was a 50 percent reduction in central line-associated bloodstream infections (CLABSIs) between 2008 and 2014, a 17 percent decrease in surgical site infections (SSIs) between 2008 and 2014, a 13 percent decrease in MRSA bacteremia between 2011 and 2014, and an 9 percent decrease in *Clostridium difficile* infections between 2011 and 2014. No change was found in the occurrence of catheter-associated urinary tract infections (CAUTIs) between 2009 and 2014.

Basic Infection Control Procedures

The WHO has issued a set of recommendations that are considered a basic standard for infection control. These guidelines aim to prevent the transmission of pathogens, including those transmitted through blood and bodily fluids. The guidelines include requirements in three key areas: hand hygiene, personal protective equipment (PPE), and respiratory hygiene and cough etiquette. In addition, the guidelines recommend that policies be developed to promote a climate of safety and to facilitate the implementation of infection control measures.

Hand hygiene is the first key to infection control because many pathogens are transmitted through direct touch or through touching a surface that another person has touched. Healthcare workers are instructed to wash their hands with soap and water for 40 to 60 seconds, using specified techniques, or (if washing with soap and water is not possible) to use an alcohol-based solution and rub their hands for 20 to 30 seconds until they are dry. Hand washing or rubbing is required before and after direct patient contact (even if gloves are used), after gloves are removed, after touching blood or bodily fluids (even if gloves are worn), before handling an invasive device, when moving from a contaminated site to a clean site (on the same patient), and after touching objects in the immediate vicinity of the patient. Operators of healthcare facilities are required to ensure that healthcare workers can follow these directions, including by providing an adequate supply of clean water, soap, alcohol-based solution, and clean towels.

PPE is the second key to infection control. Healthcare workers are expected to assess the risk of exposure to contaminated surfaces or bodily fluids and to select appropriate PPE before beginning healthcare activities. The primary types of PPE are gloves, face protection, and a gown. Gloves should be worn when touching blood, body fluids, secretions, excretions, broken skin, or mucous membranes, and should be changed between patients and between procedures on the same patient if potentially infectious material has been touched. Face protection includes a mask and eye protection, and these items should be worn as well as a gown during procedures that may create sprays or splashes of blood or other bodily fluids.

Respiratory hygiene and cough etiquette applies to visitors to healthcare facilities, as well as those who work or are cared for there. The key is that people with respiratory symptoms should wear a mask covering the nose and mouth or use a tissue to cover the nose and mouth when coughing or sneezing, then dispose of the used tissue or mask and perform appropriate hand hygiene (washing or rubbing, as detailed previously). To facilitate appropriate respiratory hygiene and cough etiquette, healthcare facilities should make supplies such as tissues, masks, and alcohol gel available in common areas, post signs instructing visitors as to appropriate hygiene measures, and if possible keep people with acute febrile respiratory symptoms at least 1 meter away from others in common areas.

Other infection control procedures apply to handling and cleaning of patient care equipment, linens, and the general environment, as well to disposal of waste. Patient care equipment should be cleaned and disinfected when moved from one patient to another. Linens should be handled in a way that avoids transfer to pathogens from a patient to the environment, other patients, or the worker. The general hospital or healthcare environment should be routinely cleaned and disinfected, with particular attention paid to frequently touched surfaces. Finally, waste items should be handled and disposed of in accordance with local regulations and in a manner that minimizes the risk of spreading infection. Human tissue and lab waste should be treated as clinical waste, as should waste contaminated with blood, body fluids, excretions, or secretions.

VACCINATION PROGRAMS

Vaccination programs are a well-known and cost-effective way to limit disease and disability worldwide. Vaccines operate by stimulating the immune system to produce antibodies that protect against specific disease, and thus may confer long-lasting disease protection. One of the most famous modern public health triumphs is the eradication of smallpox globally, due in large part to vaccination, but vaccination plays a key role in protecting individuals against many other diseases.

Vaccination programs are also relatively inexpensive in terms of the health benefits that they provide. For instance, Meghan L. Stack et al. (2011) estimate that an expanded vaccine program for children in 72 of the world's poorest countries would cost $10 billion but produce $6.2 billion in treatment savings and $145 billion in averted productivity losses. Diseases target by the vaccines in the proposed program are pneumococcal pneumonia, *Haemophilus influenzae* type b (Hib), pertussis (whooping cough), measles, rotavirus, and malaria. A separate analysis of expected benefits from the same program (Ozawa et al., 2011) estimated that the $10 billion program could provide $231 billion in savings based on the value of statistical lives saved. Many other scholars have looked at the return on investment (ROI) of vaccination programs, and most of them conclude that vaccinations are an extremely cost-effective type of healthcare intervention.

Adegbola and Saha (2010) argue that vaccination programs should be considered an important weapon in the fight against antimicrobial resistance, complementary to other programs such as the promotion of rational use of antibiotics. Vaccination programs can help reduce antibiotic use in two ways. The first is by reducing the incidence of diseases that would normally be treated by antibiotics, such as pertussis, diphtheria, and Hib pneumonia and meningitis. In addition, vaccination against viral diseases such as measles can reduce antibiotic use by reducing the risk of respiratory infections ordinarily treated with antibiotics that may follow a case of measles.

LIMITING DISEASE SPREAD THROUGH TRAVEL

The movement of human beings from one place to another has long been associated with the spread of disease. However, for much of human history, the spread of disease has been limited by the fact that travel was relatively difficult and expensive, so travel was largely limited to a few classes of people, including traders, religious pilgrims, and soldiers. By contrast, in the modern world, wide-ranging travel has become common for recreation as well as migration, employment, and religious purposes and is no longer limited to just wealthy people or residents of high-income countries. While increased mobility has brought many advantages to human society, it has also facilitated conditions in which infections can spread rapidly throughout the world. Humanitarian and military operations also result in movement of large numbers of people from one place to another, and thus may facilitate the spread of infectious disease. The conditions of travel also may facilitate the transmission of disease. Much attention has been paid, for instance, to the possibility of airborne infections being transmitted on airplanes, and of cruise ships providing excellent conditions for the spread of gastrointestinal diseases such as norovirus illness.

According to data from the Institute of Medicine, the number of international migrants (persons who have lived outside their country of birth for at least 12 months) more than doubled between 1960 and 2006, growing from 76 million to 191 million. The proportional increase was even more pronounced in the more developed regions of the world, including Europe (an increase from 14 million to 64 million over the period) and

North America (an increase from 13 million to 45 million). International tourism has also grown rapidly, with international tourist arrivals increasing from 535 million in 1995 to 846 million in 2006. As with migration, international tourists are most likely to visit European or North American countries, with the top three countries with the greatest numbers of international tourists in 2006 being France (79.1 million arrivals), Spain (58.5 million arrivals), and the United States (51.1 million arrivals). Patterns of international travel are significant in part because diseases are not uniformly spread throughout the world—for instance, tuberculosis (TB) is far more common in sub-Saharan Africa than in the United States—and international travelers may bring a disease from a region where it is common to a region where it is rare.

Efforts to limit the transmission of disease by travelers date back at least to the Middle Ages in Europe, when it was believed that the returning Crusaders introduced the plague to Europe (an account that is disputed by some present-day historians). Facilities were created to isolate and care for persons infected with leprosy, an approach to disease control that has since been applied to many other diseases. Another early infection control practice was quarantine, in which new arrivals to a city or region would be required to wait a certain length of time before being allowed to enter. The idea behind quarantine is that a person may be infected with a disease but not yet be displaying symptoms, so the quarantine period should be long enough to allow any infection to become obvious. A related measure, health inspection of arriving travelers, became common in the 19th century, with large inspection facilities created at common ports of entry such as Ellis Island and Angel Island in the United States and Grosse Ille in Canada. Some countries, including Australia, New Zealand, the United States, and Canada, continue programs of screening new immigrants for disease, although the focus has shifted from diseases like trachoma and smallpox to diseases of contemporary public health concern such as TB.

TB and Ebola

Health examinations of international travelers other than migrants is rare today. In part, this is because such measures would appear invasive to most travelers, and related measures such as quarantine in the absence of disease would be seen as a violation of individual liberties. However, screening and quarantine measures have been instituted on a short-term basis in response to outbreaks of serious disease. The possibility of serious disease being spread on an airplane was highlighted by a 2007 case in the United States, in which an individual, Andrew Speaker, infected with multi-drug-resistant TB (MDR-TB) flew from the United States to France, Greece, and Italy, and returned on a flight from the Czech Republic to Canada, reentering the United States by driving over the border. At the time, it was believed that Speaker was infected with a more serious disease, extensively drug-resistant TB (XDR-TB), which heightened public concern about the ease with which an infected individual could travel by air, possibly endangering the health of other passengers and the flight crew, as well as the people living in the countries he visited.

In 2014, a serious outbreak of Ebola in several West African countries prompted some countries to restrict the entry of travelers from countries where Ebola was present, institute medical screening procedures for travelers arriving from those countries, or both. Exit screening (for travelers leaving the county) was also instituted at airports in the countries where Ebola was epidemic. Typical elements of an exit screening include answering questions about exposure to Ebola and having one's temperature taken (fever is associated with Ebola infection). However, neither procedure is foolproof because individuals may not know that they have been exposed, or they may lie about it, and temperature measurements can be inaccurate. In addition, a person may be carrying the virus but not yet have developed a fever or other symptoms.

The Ebola outbreak also caused the United States to apply two public health measures: contact tracing and monitoring of potentially exposed persons. The first confirmed case of Ebola in the United States (the index case) was identified on September 30, 2014. The patient had been in Liberia and did not have symptoms when he left that country, but became ill after returning to the United States, demonstrating the limitations of screening programs. Close contacts of the patient were contacted by public health officials and monitored for 21 days, and none became ill with the disease. Despite the use of strenuous infection control procedures, two healthcare workers who cared for the infected patient also became infected. One of these healthcare workers had traveled on two airplane flights after exposure to the patient, and all the passengers and crew on both flights were contacted by public health officials and required to undergo a 21-day monitoring period. The fourth known case of Ebola in the United States was identified on October 23, 2014, in an individual who had been serving with Doctors Without Borders in Guinea.

Although no national quarantine was imposed in the United States following the Ebola outbreak in West Africa, several states, including New York, New Jersey, Connecticut, and California, imposed mandatory 21-day quarantines for persons exposed to Ebola. Other states, including Maine,

Florida, Georgia, Maryland, and Pennsylvania, imposed mandatory surveillance procedures, such as temperature reporting, for individuals exposed to Ebola.

DEVELOPING NEW ANTIBIOTICS AND IMPROVED DIAGNOSTIC TESTS

New antibiotics for human use are discovered and refined through a combination of lab research and clinical trials, and the process to develop a new drug is time consuming and expensive. While many new antibiotics, many of which were effective against many types of bacteria, were developed in the early years of the antibiotics era (from the 1940s through the 1950s, sometimes referred to as "the golden age of antibiotics discovery"), fewer have come from the drug development process in recent years. Even in the past few decades, the number of new antibiotics approved for use in the United States has dropped, from almost 20 in 1980–1984 to only 2 in 2010–2012. Because bacteria naturally develop resistance to the antibiotics used against them, one important way to fight drug resistance is to develop new drugs to which the bacteria are not resistant.

Several reasons have been offered for the slowing in the discovery of new antibiotics. One is that the earliest antibiotics (e.g., penicillin and tetracycline) could be considered "low-hanging fruit" that were relatively easy to discover and develop, whereas the discovery and development of new antibiotics that can treat microbes resistant to previously discovered drugs is more difficult and time consuming. For instance, a 2008 study found that of 167 antibiotics under development, only 15 were likely to prove useful in treating MDR bacteria.

Another is that the development of antimicrobials does not provide the greatest ROI for pharmaceutical companies because most antibiotics are taken by an individual for only a short period of time. In contrast, drugs used to treat chronic diseases or conditions such as diabetes or high blood pressure may be taken by the same patient for years, resulting in higher sales of such drugs. As of 2008, only five major pharmaceutical companies— AstraZeneca, GlaxoSmithKline, Merck, Novartis, and Pfizer—had active antibacterial discovery programs.

Another reason that it is important to be researching new types of antibiotics constantly is because the drugs that have been approved may be unsuitable for some patients or have side effects that make them a less desirable treatment. For instance, televancin, which is effective against *Staphylococcus*, *Streptococcus*, and *Enterococcus* infections, cannot be used during pregnancy. In addition, this drug must be administered intravenously, making it inconvenient for administration outside a hospital setting.

SURVEILLANCE AND REPORTING PROGRAMS

Public health surveillance plays an important role in the fight against drug resistance. According to the WHO, this surveillance should be continuous and systematic and involve analysis and interpretation, as well as the collection of data that can be used in planning, implementing, and evaluating public health practice. An effective surveillance program collects data over a period of time in a way that allows public health officials to notice changes in the health of a population or factors that affect the health of a population over time. Effective surveillance can alert officials to impending public health emergency, track progress toward public health goals, and aid in evaluating the impact of interventions and developing health policies and setting priorities in public health programs.

While public health professionals understand the importance of surveillance programs, they are expensive and generally require funding from government sources. Because every government has to meet multiple demands for services with limited funds, it may be difficult for those involved in public health surveillance to convince public officials to provide sufficient funding for their programs. This can lead to gaps in information, which in turn can make it difficult or impossible for officials to track changes in disease trends, including antibiotic resistance, evaluate how well interventions are working, or identify new threats to public health. However, because many of these benefits are only seen over time, as opposed to the direct delivery of services (e.g., paying for health clinics), those involved in public health may have particular difficulties in obtaining adequate funding.

Public health surveillance also requires coordination among people working in different regions and in different levels of government (local, regional, national, and international), and different priorities and local cultures may compound difficulties in carrying out surveillance programs. Much of the data needed for public health surveillance must be collected at the local level, even if it may be aggregated and analyzed at the regional or national level—the initial work of collecting local data cannot be done long distance. Unfortunately, not all countries have sufficient resources, in terms of money and trained personnel, to conduct effective surveillance programs, so organizations like the WHO often help develop and operate effective surveillance programs in developing countries. Further, although data analyses at the national level are useful in helping understand the scope of drug resistance, analyses at the international level are also required, and this responsibility has fallen largely to international organizations and researchers in industrialized countries.

Tracking Antimicrobial Resistance in the United States

In the United States, the CDC is engaged in multiple efforts to gather data on antimicrobial resistance. While the CDC's methods may not be applicable to every country because surveillance must be appropriate to local conditions and resources, they are worth elaborating on because they demonstrate how complex the process of tracking antimicrobial resistance can be. The CDC gathers data through five tracking programs: the NHSN, the Emerging Infections Program (EIP), the National Antimicrobial Resistance Monitoring System (NARMS), the Gonococcal Isolate Surveillance Program (GISP), and the National Tuberculosis Surveillance Program (NTSS).

The EIP consists of three programs: Active Bacterial Core (ABC) surveillance, the Healthcare-Associated Infections Community Interface (HAIC), and the Foodborne Diseases Active Surveillance Network (FoodNet). ABCs collects clinical information and resistance data for the bacterias *Streptococcus pneumoniae*, *Streptococccus* Groups A and B, methicillin-resistant *Staphylococcus aureus* (MRSA), and the viruses *Neisseria meningitidis* and *Haemophilus influenzae*, all of which cause infections primarily in the community (as opposed to in healthcare settings). The HAIC collects clinical information and resistance data on the bacterias *C. difficile*, carbapenem-resistant *Enterobacteriaceae*, MDR *Acinetobacter*, and the fungus *Candida*, all of which cause infections at the intersection of the community and the healthcare system. FoodNet collects clinical and epidemiologic data on human isolates of the bacterias *Salmonella*, *Campylobacter*, and *Shigella*.

NARMS is a collaboration of three national agencies: the CDC, the U.S. Food and Drug Administration (FDA), the U.S. Department of Agriculture (USDA), and health departments at the state and local levels. All three collect information on the bacterias *Salmonella*, *Campylobacter*, *Shigella*, *E. coli O157*, and *Vibrio* (*non-V. cholerae*), and track changes in the susceptibility of enteric bacteria, including foodborne bacteria, to antibiotics. The CDC studies bacterial isolates from humans, while the FDA and USDA test isolates from food animals and retail meats.

The GISP tracks antibiotic resistance for *N. gonorrhoeae*, collecting information on gonococcal isolates collected from clinics treating sexually transmitted diseases (STDs) in a number of cities (28 cities as of 2013). The NTSS collects information about *Mycobacterium* TB through the National

Electronic Disease Surveillance System (NEDSS), which gathers information from public health departments in all U.S. states and territories regarding TB cases and drug resistance.

Tracking Antimicrobial Resistance Globally

The WHO produced its first global report on antimicrobial resistance surveillance in 2014. This report, *Antimicrobial Resistance: Global Report on Surveillance 2014*, identified several key gaps in surveillance. Because of these gaps, it is difficult to know the true scope of the problem of antimicrobial resistance or to plan effective strategies to deal with it.

The first gap comes from the lack of standardized procedures and tools to collect information about antimicrobial resistance, including its current level and consequences in both humans and animals. In addition, better integration is needed among efforts to track antimicrobial resistance in all levels of the food chain. Finally, systems for population-based surveillance of antimicrobial resistance need to be established in the countries that do not already have such systems, in order to ensure that information about antimicrobial resistance represents the situation in the entire country.

Despite these shortcomings (which are not surprising given that surveillance of antimicrobial resistance has been carried out largely on a country level rather than an international level, and given that different countries have vastly different levels of resources to dedicate to the effort), the WHO reached several conclusions. One is that antimicrobial resistance is a widespread problem, and that in some parts of the world, many standard treatment options for common diseases are no longer effective. The second conclusion is that antimicrobial resistance results in increased expenditures for healthcare and worse outcomes for patients. The third conclusion is that surveillance programs are best established for drugs used to treat TB, malaria, and HIV, and that lessons learned from successful programs in those areas can be applied to surveillance of antimicrobial resistance for drugs used to treat other diseases.

RECOMMENDATIONS FOR GLOBAL SURVEILLANCE

The Review on Antimicrobial Resistance, an independent organization commissioned by the prime minister of the United Kingdom and the Wellcome Trust, offers three suggestions for actions that would help to develop globally integrated systems surveillance of drug resistance. The first is to provide more funding for such efforts and to better coordinate current and new surveillance efforts. The need for greater funding is obvious, particularly in low-income countries where better infrastructure must be developed and personnel trained to do the work of surveillance and analysis. Because it will take time to develop a globally integrated system of surveillance, the review recommends that smaller studies (e.g., measuring the prevalence of drug-resistant bacteria at a single location) should continue while the globally integrated system is being developed.

The second action recommended is to address the problems inherent in any project when data are collected and combined from many sources. These issues include lack of common standards for data collection and dissemination, concerns about patient confidentiality and the level of data aggregation, differing ideas about who owns data and how they can be used, inconsistent data collection protocols, and concerns about data quality. These issues are technical but require consensus at the international level in order to facilitate data sharing and analysis.

The third action recommended is that privately held data (e.g., that collected by a private health insurer or pharmacy benefit management company) should become part of national and global surveillance systems. This would be beneficial because in many countries, a large proportion of healthcare services are provided by private entities, and any analysis based only on public healthcare providers thus must be incomplete and may be misleading. One key challenge in taking this action is resolving the issue of who has the right to data that have been collected by a private (often for-profit) entity, but which are essential to address issues of public health. When data will be shared on an international level, additional concerns about confidentiality and intellectual property rights are also heightened.

Contemporary Issues and Debates

Drug Resistance as a National and International Issue

Often, we think of health issues at a local or individual level, with the most obvious case being, in the case of medicine, one physician treating one patient. Of course, it is important to focus on this aspect of medical practice—when you are the patient, your own health is your primary concern, and when a physician treats a patient, the welfare of that patient is also the physician's primary concern—but some issues of health demand consideration of a context larger than the relationship between two individuals. This is recognized in the field of public health, where regulations safeguarding the safety of the municipal water supply and requiring that children receive certain immunizations before attending school are intended to improve the health of many individuals.

Such practices and regulations are based in part on the reality that one person's actions may affect the life of other people, even without that intention on the part of the actor. For instance, if someone pollutes the water supply for a city, the health of everyone who depends on that source for clean drinking water may be endangered. Similarly, a person who is not immunized and contracts a disease or becomes a carrier of a disease can pass it on to others. Conversely, people can benefit from practices of which they are unaware. In many countries, provision of clean drinking water is assumed, and an individual consuming water safeguarded through that system benefits from lack of exposure to waterborne disease even if they are unaware of the system. Similarly, if a high proportion of a population (the specific proportion required varies from one disease to another) is immune to a disease, whether through immunization or from having the disease, even people who are not immunized are protected from the disease due to *herd immunity* (also known as *community immunity*).

Mass immunization programs are based in part on this concept of herd immunity. Often, not everyone in a society can receive an immunization due to compromised immune system, very young age, or some other reason. If a sufficient proportion of the population is immunized, however, it greatly reduces the risk of nonimmunized individuals being exposed to the disease that the immunization is meant to prevent. High rates of immunization also limit the spread of the disease (so that a single case is unlikely to lead to an outbreak or epidemic), and in the best-case situation, they can lead to the eradication of a disease (meaning that it no longer exists among the human population, so no one is at risk of contracting it). As with clean water, an individual can benefit from herd immunity without even being aware of it.

While the use of medications has largely been viewed as an individual decision or a decision to be made by a physician and patient together, a broader context is also relevant in at least some cases. The use of antibiotics is one of those cases because the overuse or misuse of antibiotics encourages the development and growth of drug-resistant strains of diseases that can infect other people. Needless to say, microbes observe no political boundaries, and with modern systems of transportation, a microbe originating in one area may quickly spread to other parts of the world, infecting people far from the location of the original patient. For this reason, the fight against drug resistance is conducted at multiple levels, from the local to the international level.

STAKEHOLDERS

Many different parties are stakeholders in the use of antibiotics, and sometimes their interests are not aligned with each other. For instance, an ill patient understandably wants to get better and may be less concerned about the effect of their behavior on the health of others; this attitude can lead to the overuse or misuse of antibiotics. No one expects patients to have a medical education, so a person with a viral infection may believe that antibiotics will help cure his or her disease. In addition, individual patients may not understand the harm of taking an unneeded antibiotic and may feel "better safe than sorry" when trying to improve their own health.

A physician wants to cure his or her patient and also wants the patient to be satisfied with the care received. Those desires may also lead to the overprescription of an antibiotic, perhaps because the patient wants it and the physician prefers to write a prescription, even if the prescribed drug is unlikely to help the patient, rather than have the patient be upset. In addition, patients may go from one doctor to another until they find one that will pre-scribe the desired antibiotics.

In the case of individual patients and physicians, national and interna-tional organizations can play a key role in limiting the inappropriate use of antibiotics by educating individuals as to the potential harm of antibiotic overuse and the lack of benefit to patients when antibiotics are used to treat diseases for which they are not effective. Because large organizations stand outside the interest of either party, they can speak with greater impartiality about the appropriate use of antibiotics. The reputation and prestige of such organizations, particularly if they are trusted to make recommendations based on science rather than profit or other motives, also may make their recommendations more likely to be followed.

Pharmaceutical companies produce medicines that can save lives, includ-ing antibiotics. However, like other for-profit companies, they have incen-tives to reduce their own costs in ways that do not limit their ability to make their products. One way to cut costs is through improper disposal of waste, and in the case of antibiotics, this can lead to the development of resistance. For instance, Kristiansson et al. (2011) found high concentrations of bacte-ria containing resistance genes and other elements promoting drug resistance in river soil downstream of antibiotic production plants. They also found high levels of antibiotics in the water itself—sometimes at a concentration equivalent to a therapeutic dose—so the polluted water was essentially releasing doses of antibiotics into the environment. The research of Kris-tiansson and colleagues was based on analysis of conditions near Hyder-abad, India, and they determined that the water containing antibiotics came from nearby bulk pharmaceutical manufacturers. However, other studies have found high levels of pharmaceuticals in waters surrounding drug-manufacturing plants, including plants in the United States, so this problem may be more widespread than is currently believed. While issues of pollu-tion are often handled at the local or national level, the fact that resistant genes can be spread throughout the world means that international organ-izations also have an interest in identifying practices that can lead to the development of antibiotic resistance.

RECOMMENDATIONS FOR ANTIBIOTIC USE

International Recommendations

No organization has the power to regulate antibiotic use at the interna-tional level. However, international organizations can play an important role in encouraging the appropriate use of antibiotics, conducting research and developing tools to collect data about antibiotic use and antimicrobial resistance, facilitating efforts of national and regional organizations to create and implement policies governing the use of antibiotics, and coordinating the collection and sharing of data regarding antimicrobial use and antimicrobial resistance.

For instance, the World Health Organization (WHO) has created guidelines and recommendations for antibiotic use that may influence prescribing practices and other aspects of antibiotic use in many countries. Other international organizations may also create such guidelines and recommendations. The WHO and other international organizations generally lack direct enforcement power to lack the power to enforce these standards directly because they do not have that authority, and any attempt by WHO to interfere in the relationship between a physician and patient would be seen as overreaching by many people. However, by publicizing recommendations for best practices, promoting scientific research into issues related to antibiotic resistance, and providing public and professional education regarding antibiotic use and the consequences of antibiotic resistance, the WHO and other international organizations can indirectly influence the way that antibiotics are throughout the world.

In 2014, the WHO published *Antimicrobial Resistance: Global Report on Surveillance*, the first attempt to address the problem of drug resistance and the state of information and surveillance systems by gathering data about drug resistance on a global basis. The report concentrates on drug-resistant microbes, particularly bacteria, responsible for common infections in both healthcare and community settings, including tuberculosis (TB), malaria, pneumonia, dysentery, gonorrhea, and urinary tract infections (UTIs). The report also found serious gaps in surveillance programs for antimicrobial resistance and concluded that antimicrobial resistance is a global threat to health and that gaps in surveillance programs hamper efforts to address the issue.

Antimicrobial Resistance also states that the WHO will play a role in addressing these issues by acting as a source of expertise and facilitating coordination of surveillance efforts and information sharing throughout the world. Three specific ways that the WHO plans to aid in improving global surveillance of antimicrobial resistance are listed in the report, as follows:

1. Helping to develop tools and standards for surveillance, and for integrating surveillance efforts in human and animal populations
2. Facilitating the elaboration of strategies for population-based surveillance of antimicrobial resistance and its impact on health and on the economy

DRUG RESISTANCE AS A NATIONAL AND INTERNATIONAL ISSUE   83

3. Aiding collaboration between surveillance networks and centers and between global and regional surveillance programs.

On May 24, 2014, the Sixty-seventh World Health Assembly (the governing body of the WHO) issued Resolution WAH 67.25, "Antimicrobial Resistance." This resolution affirms the leadership role of the WHO in the fight against antimicrobial resistance, as well as the importance of preventing the growth of antimicrobial resistance for both health and economic reasons. It also recognized the establishment of the WHO Global Task Force on Antimicrobial Resistance and the collaboration between the WHO, the Food and Agriculture Organization of the United Nations (FAO), and the World Organisation for Animal Health (OIE, or *Organisation mondiale de la santé animale*) in addressing this issue.

This resolution contains two sections calling for action: one addressed to member-states of the WHO and one to the director-general of the WHO. The choice of language in both cases is significant: member-states are *urged*, and the director-general is *requested*, to undertake certain actions. This choice of language underlines the fact that the WHO has no power to enforce these requests, but as a leader in international health, it is recommending that actions be taken by the governments of the member-states and by the leader of the WHO.

The resolution makes 10 recommendations for member-states:

1. Increase efforts to promote appropriate antimicrobial use
2. Strengthen infection control measures
3. Create or strengthen national strategies and international collaborations focused on the containment of antimicrobial resistance
4. Implement plans and strategies to contain antimicrobial resistance
5. Strengthen pharmaceutical management systems to ensure that effective antimicrobial agents are available to those who need them
6. Monitor antibiotic use and antimicrobial resistance, and share that information
7. Increase awareness of the dangers posed by antimicrobial resistance, the need to use antibiotics responsibly, and the importance of infection control
8. Support research and development to combat antimicrobial resistance
9. Help develop, in collaboration with the World Health Organization, a global action plan to help combat antimicrobial resistance

10. Develop surveillance systems for antimicrobial resistance in hospitals, outpatient care settings, and in animal husbandry and other non-human settings

The requests to the director are statements of actions to be taken by the leader of the WHO, which identify the organization's priorities in the fight against antimicrobial resistance. Seven requests are included:

1. Ensure that the World Health Organization is engaged in combating antimicrobial resistance, and coordinates work carried out at the headquarters, regional, and country levels
2. Allocate adequate resources for this work
3. Strengthen collaboration to combat antimicrobial resistance among the WHO, the Food and Agriculture Organization (FAO) of the United Nations, and the World Organisation for Animal Health (OIE)
4. Explore options for collaboration with the United Nations to combat antimicrobial resistance
5. Develop a draft global action plan to combat antimicrobial resistance that takes into account existing programs and scientific evidence, and that addresses the need for adequate resources in low- and middle-income countries to address this problem
6. Consult member-states and other relevant stakeholders while creating the global action plan
7. Submit this global action plan at the Sixty-eighth World Health Assembly

National Recommendations in the United States

In the United States, antibiotics are available only by prescription. One reason for this restriction is that untrained individuals are unlikely to be able to determine when an illness would be helped by taking an antibiotic and when it would not. For instance, a sore throat caused by a virus, which would not be affected by antibiotics, may feel very much like a sore throat caused by the *Streptococcus* bacteria, which can be treated successfully by antibiotics. If antibiotics were freely available over the counter (i.e., without presentation of a prescription by a physician or someone else with prescribing authority, such as a nurse practitioner), many people might purchase and consume antibiotics in response to symptoms caused by viruses or other agents not susceptible to antibiotics, one of the practices that help create antibiotic-resistant strains of bacteria.

While there is no national governing body with the power to regulate how antibiotics are prescribed by physicians (which would be considered an intrusion into the doctor-patient relationship), several professional organizations and government agencies have created guidelines for appropriate antibiotic use, as well as educational materials for both health professionals and the general public concerning antibiotics, their appropriate use, and the dangers of antibiotic resistance.

The Centers of Disease Control and Prevention (CDC), part of the National Institutes of Health (NIH) within the U.S. Department of Health and Human Services, has issued guidelines for antibiotic prescribing and created educational materials relating to antibiotics use. For instance, the March 2014 issue of *CDC Vital Signs*, a publication of the CDC, contains information about antibiotic use in hospitals, the risks of overprescribing antibiotics, recommendations for action by several types of stakeholders to help curb the overuse of antibiotics, and specific recommendations for prescribing practices in hospitals. The issue also includes links to more information about these issues and examples of programs that have improved antibiotic-prescribing practices.

Although the CDC does not have the power to enforce these recommendations, they carry weight because this organization is respected as a leader in the field of public health and a reliable source of medical and public health information. The CDC recommendations recognize that there are many different stakeholders in healthcare who may influence antibiotic-prescribing practices, and that the complex ways that healthcare is provided, regulated, and paid for in the United States mean that the problems must be addressed at numerous levels. Given this understanding, the CDC makes specific recommendations for the federal government, state and local health departments, hospital chief executive officers (CEOs) and medical officers, doctors and other hospital staff, and hospital patients, each of which can play a role in improving antibiotic use and lowering the threat of antibiotic resistance.

The CDC makes six recommendations for action by the federal government:

1. Help hospitals track antibiotic use and resistance by expanding the National Healthcare Safety Network
2. Share recommendations and tools intended to improve prescribing practices with clinicians and administrators
3. Support the testing of ways to improve prescribing practices
4. Help create regional programs to improve prescribing practices

5. Create an antibiotic stewardship program for Veterans Administration hospitals
6. Provide incentives for the development of new antibiotics

The CDC recommends that state and local health departments do the following:

1. Learn about local antibiotic stewardship activities
2. Facilitate efforts to improve prescribe practices and prevent antibiotic resistance
3. Provide physicians with educational tools to improve prescribing practices

Recommendations for hospital CEOs and medical officers are that they, at a minimum:

1. Commit the necessary resources to the antibiotic stewardship program
2. Appoint a single leader responsible for the program's outcomes
3. Appoint a single pharmacist leader to the program
4. Take at least one action toward improving prescribing practice
5. Monitor prescribing practices and antibiotic resistance patterns
6. Report prescribing practices and antibiotic resistance patterns to staff members
7. Offer educational programs concerning antibiotic-prescribing practices and antibiotic resistance

The CDC makes five recommendations for physicians and hospital staff:

1. Follow correct antibiotics-prescribing practices
2. Document the indication, dose, and duration for every antibiotic prescription
3. Be aware of antibiotic-resistance practices within the hospital
4. Lead and take part in efforts to improve prescribing practices within the hospital
5. Follow infection control procedures, including hand hygiene

Finally, the CDC offers two recommendations for patients:

1. Ask if tests will be done to ensure use of the correct antibiotic
2. Be sure that staff clean their hands before touching you, and if you have a catheter, ask every day if it is necessary that you continue using it.

The CDC offers three general guidelines for antibiotics-prescribing in hospitals and specific recommendations for three common diseases: UTIs, pneumonia, and methicillin-resistant *Staphylococcus aureus* (MRSA) infections. The general guidelines are:

1. Order recommended cultures before prescribing antibiotics, and begin drug treatment promptly if warranted
2. Include indication, dose, and expected duration of treatment in the patient record
3. Reassess prescriptions within 24 hours and adjust or halt treatment if indicated.

The strong point of the CDC recommendations may be their awareness of the complex nature of medical care and of the many different stakeholders that may influence antibiotic use in hospitals. Many recommendations are obvious (e.g., documenting prescriptions and following recommended prescribing practices) and, at least theoretically, are already being followed, but others are impractical and ignore the practicalities of how a hospital functions. For instance, patients who ask every day if a catheter is necessary or question how the drugs prescribed for them were chosen may be considered a nuisance by hospital staff. Similarly, programs to track antibiotic resistance and educate staff cost money that may not be available in a hospital budget.

DEVELOPING NEW ANTIBIOTICS

The antibiotic revolution of the mid-20th century was possible because of the discovery of new drugs such as penicillin and streptomycin, which were rightly hailed as "miracle drugs" when first introduced into medical practice. These drugs could treat, and often cure, common diseases, some of them potentially fatal, for which medical science had had little to offer in the way of effective treatment. The period from the 1930s through the 1950s was marked by the introduction of many important classes of antibiotics, including sulfa drugs, several types of penicillin, aminoglycosides (including streptomycin), tetracyclines, macrolides (including erythromycin), and tetracyclines (including streptomycin, tetracycline, neomycin, and vancomycin).

The success of these drugs in conquering or limiting the harm caused by previously common infections led to less research being devoted to developing new antibiotics, and consequently fewer new antibiotics being brought to market. For instance, in the period 1983 to 1987, 16 new antibiotics were approved for use in the United States; by 2008 to 2011, this number had fallen to only 2 new antibiotics approved, or less than 1 per year. As the growth of antibiotic resistance has made many formerly effective antibiotics less useful in fighting disease, attention has shifted once again to the need for continuing investment in research and development to find new antibiotics and classes of antibiotics.

New Drug Development

Pharmaceutical research and development is an international industry, with key players including the United States, the United Kingdom, Switzerland, and France. Notably, these are all high-income countries, which is not surprising: Most pharmaceutical research and development is conducted in industrialized countries and is mostly privately financed, rather than being funded by governments or by nonprofits. In contrast, the toll of death and disability caused by infectious diseases is most severe in developing countries. Many scholars see these circumstances as one reason why research and development of new antibiotics has declined: companies have little incentive to invest in the research and development of antibiotics that are not a major concern to people in the countries that they see as their most important markets. One figure, cited in a 2014 report to the president of the United States by the President's Council of Advisors on Science and Technology, said that fewer than 10 percent of the top 50 pharmaceutical companies worldwide have active programs of antibiotic development.

There is no question that the drug development process is long and costly and that the number of new drugs introduced to the market each year is a small fraction of those initially considered worthy of study. For instance, according to the FDA, the agency responsible for governing the drug approval process in the United States, for every drug that is successfully brought to market, another 5,000 to 10,000 substances were considered potentially useful but did not make it through the review process. The process of bringing a new drug to market can take 10 to 15 years and cost as much as $1 billion. There is a general consensus that developing a new drug is an expensive and risky endeavor and that most attempts to develop novel compounds that will result in bringing a new drug to market will not succeed.

Pharmaceutical companies may produce lifesaving medications, but like other for-profit companies, they must also make a profit to survive. While the pharmaceutical industry has been criticized for producing too many "me too" drugs, which treat conditions for which adequate therapies are already available, this criticism ignores the fact that pharmaceutical companies are for-profit entities, not public charities. It is an arguable point whether our current model of pharmaceutical research and development is the best possible way to get this work done, but it is the system we have and the context in which most drugs are developed and brought to market.

Besides the fact that the need for new antibiotics is greatest in developing countries, which comprise a small fraction of the world pharmaceuticals market, another factor that may discourage companies from investing in developing new antibiotics is that most are taken for only a brief period (e.g., 10 days), as compared to drugs to treat chronic conditions such as high cholesterol or high blood pressure, which may be taken for years or decades. On average, there is more money to be made selling a drug that must be taken over a long period of time, and that treats a disease common in high-income countries, than in developing a drug that can cure a disease in a short period of time and that is used primarily to treat diseases prevalent in low-income countries.

Efforts to Increase Antibiotics Research and Development

Recognizing that private companies, which currently perform most pharmaceutical research and development, do not have sufficient financial incentive to research new antibiotics in current market conditions, alternative ways to develop new drugs have been suggested. This is a complex process because of the large numbers of stakeholders involved, the high cost of developing any new drug, and the need to balance competing priorities.

One competing pair of priorities is the need for drugs to address health needs versus the need for commercial companies to make a profit (or to maximize revenue). The purpose of these new initiatives is not to destroy existing pharmaceutical companies, but to create alternative paths to development or alternative incentives within the current structure that will foster the creation of new antibiotics. Another competing pair of priorities is the need for new drugs to treat drug-resistant infections while also ensuring that any new drug brought to market is safe and effective. While there is an urgent need for new, effective antibiotics to treat drug-resistant infections, no one wants to see a recurrence of, say, the thalidomide episode of the 1950s and early 1960s, when thousands of children suffered severe birth defects due to prenatal exposure to this drug (mainly in Europe, as this drug was never approved for use in the United States).

Europe

One initiative aimed at developing drugs to meet unmet needs, including treating antibiotic-resistant infections, is the Innovative Medicines Initiative (IMI), launched in 2008. The IMI is a joint undertaking of the European Union (EU) and the European Federation of Pharmaceutical Industries and Associations (EFPIA), an organization that includes 33 national

pharmaceutical industry associations in Europe and 40 countries perform-
ing research, development, and manufacture of pharmaceuticals in Europe.

The mission of the IMI is to speed up the development of innovative
medicines, particularly those relevant to areas in which there is an unmet
medical or social need, and to improve patient access to those medicines.
The budget for the IMI is 3.3 billion euros for the period 2014–2024, making
it the largest public-private life sciences partnership in the world. As of
2015, the IMI has over 50 projects underway, including DRIVE-AB, a project devoted to addressing a fundamental paradox in antibiotic development
and use. The world needs new antibiotics to treat drug-resistant infections,
but the use of antibiotics must be restricted to slow the development of resistance. Because of this paradox, antibiotics carry a lower return on investment
(ROI) than many other types of drugs, and thus pharmaceutical companies
are less inclined to focus their funds on antibiotic development.

DRIVE-AB is focused on the economic aspects of antibiotic development and use and is devoted to developing recommendations for economic
models to provide the pharmaceutical industry with an incentive to invest
in the development of new antibiotics, while at the same time promoting the
safe use of antibiotics. This project is currently slated to run from 2014
through 2017, including a team of experts drawn from both academia and
the pharmaceutical industry.

The final goal of DRIVE-AB is to develop an economic model that provides adequate incentives for both the development of new antibiotics and
their responsible use. This process begins with developing a consensus-
based definition of responsible antibiotic use and estimation of the current
burden of antibiotic resistance based on data and previous scientific research.
The team then will develop an estimate of the true value of new and existing antibiotics and develop reward models and economic strategies that will
meet three goals: fostering the development of new antibiotics, promoting
the responsible use of antibiotics, and ensuring that antibiotics are available to patients who need them.

United States

In the United States, several different strategies have been proposed to
foster the development of new antibiotics. One is to increase government
funding for research focused on developing new antibiotics for human use.
For instance, the 2014 report by the President's Council of Advisors on
Science and Technology suggested that the federal government should
devote $150 million per year for seven years to supporting antibiotic
research, primarily through the NIH and the FDA. The same report suggests

establishing a national clinical trial network to help speed up the clinical trials process for antibiotics, and to provide $25 million annually in funding to create and support the infrastructure necessary for such a network.

A second proposal is to create a dedicated clinical trial network for antibiotics in order to accommodate several peculiarities of antibiotic use. First, antibiotics are often used to treat acute infections, and thus a physician's first priority is to get an effective treatment to patients rather than delaying the process to allow them to enroll in a clinical trial. A second problem is that any clinical trial site may have only a few patients eligible to enroll at any given time because unlike chronic diseases, the infections treated by antibiotics are often of short duration. Third, the current process of conducting drug trials through pharmaceutical companies means that each company creates its own network of trial sites, a slow and inefficient process. By creating a national network, it is hoped that patients could be enrolled rapidly, from sites all over the country, and without needing to rely on existing networks established by pharmaceutical manufacturers.

A third proposal to foster the development of new antibiotics suggests creating a new pathway that would speed up the process of bringing a new drug to market. Such a pathway could allow a drug to be tested in a smaller and more focused population than is normally required by the FDA, and allow a drug to be approved to treat only antibiotic-resistant infections rather than all infections caused by a specific microbe.

The creation of a special pathway to initial FDA approval was suggested in a 2012 report by the President's Council of Advisors on Science and Technology. This "special medical use (SMU)" pathway would allow the FDA to grant initial approval to a drug when a clinical trial had been conducted in a limited and defined group of patients and was demonstrated to be safe and effective within that population, and would allow drugs to become available without having gone through clinical trials with the broader populations usually required for FDA trials. In addition, a drug approved through the SMU pathway would be recommended for use only when existing antibiotics were unable to treat an infection, thus limiting its use and hopefully slowing the development of resistance to the new drug.

Limiting the use of an approved drug would be problematic in the United States because physicians are generally allowed to prescribe FDA-approved drugs for off-label use (i.e., for uses other than those for which the drug is specifically recommended). However, the FDA can provide physician education and other procedures such as the use of warning labels to discourage the use of SMU-approved drugs for infections that could be treated by other antibiotics already in common use.

The report to the president also proposed four methods to address the conflict, also highlighted by the IMI, between the need for new antibiotics and classes of antibiotics, as well as the fact that the pharmaceutical industry can make greater profits by focusing on other types of drugs. None of these methods would be easy to implement, requiring substantial governmental expenditures and possibly new legislation to implement, and also might be politically unpopular. However, the report argues that antibiotic development should be regarded as a public good, and thus is a legitimate use of public funds.

One possibility is to provide public funds directly to support the research into and development of new types of antibiotics, an approach known as a "push" mechanism. This type of funding is already in use in the United States: For instance, the Biomedical Advanced Research and Development Authority (BARDA), part of the U.S. Department of Health and Human Services, provides funding and promotes research partnerships to develop countermeasures against bioterrorism threats. These threats include emerging infectious diseases and pandemic influenza, as well as chemical, biological, radiological, and nuclear dangers. BARDA includes an antibiotic development partnership that typically requires that half the funding for a project to develop a new drug be provided by the company doing the development, with the other half provided as public funds through BARDA.

A second way that the government can promote the development of new antibiotics is through "pull" mechanisms, which increase the economic rewards that companies can expect to receive after a new drug is approved. The concept behind pull mechanisms is that with a higher reward available for a successful new drug, companies will be more motivated to invest their own funds in the drug development process. One way to provide this type of incentive is by providing more reimbursement for new antibiotics, such as by increasing the premium allowed for reimbursement through the Centers for Medicare and Medicaid Services. This type of incentive is easily implemented, but it is unclear how much of an incentive would be needed to encourage companies to undergo the risk and expense of developing antibiotics.

A third way that the government could promote the development of new antibiotics is to provide a payment to a manufacturer for developing a new antibiotic independent of its use, such as by awarding a lump-sum prize when the drug is approved. Similar results could be achieved by having the government buy the patent for an important new drug from the company that developed it. In either case, this method has the beneficial effect of reversing the linkage of payments and usage, a practice that encourages companies to promote the sale of their drugs and that can result in the overuse of antibiotics and the creation of conditions favoring the development of antibiotic resistance.

A fourth method is to extend the patent period for new antibiotics, thus granting market exclusivity for a longer time and presumably increasing the profits made from the new drug. This would delay the transition of a new drug to generic status, and thus probably mean that it would carry a higher price. In some proposals, the company developing an important new antibiotic would be provided with a voucher to extend the market exclusivity of any drug, and the company could sell that voucher to another company to be applied to a different drug.

CHAPTER 7

Changing Physician and Pharmacist Behavior

In many countries, access to antibiotics is restricted by law. In some, a patient must present a prescription from a physician or other medical professional before being allowed to purchase such a drug. In other countries, pharmacists are allowed to dispense antibiotics based on their professional judgment of a patient's needs. Physicians, pharmacists, and other professionals with prescribing privileges (such as nurse practitioners in the United States) are assumed to have sufficient knowledge and experience to determine when patients would benefit by taking antibiotics and when they would not. Nevertheless, many studies have found that antibiotics are often prescribed inappropriately, and for that reason, one aspect of slowing the growth of antibiotic resistance is promoting responsible antibiotic-prescribing practices.

Because of the intimate and privileged nature of the physician-patient relationship, most proposals to promote the appropriate use of antibiotics in medicine and to curb the inappropriate use focus on education rather than regulation or prohibition. This is particularly true in countries such as the United States, where health is considered primarily an individual concern; in other countries, the public health aspect of medicine is given a relatively higher priority. Even in countries where health is conceived of primarily on an individual basis, however, the threat of antibiotic resistance, which could affect any individual, has led to a greater focus on creating standards for antibiotic use and educating physicians and other prescribers in the rational use of antibiotics.

Decision Making in Medicine

Viewed from the outside, medical decision making may seem to be a simple process. The patient shows up with an illness, the physician conducts an interview and conducts tests, diagnoses the illness, and writes a prescription for a drug to cure it. This misleading view of the medical decision-making process may be due in part to television programs in which physicians rapidly make the correct diagnosis of even the most baffling illness and prescribe effective treatments just as easily. It also may be because most people experience medicine only as a patient, and thus are not aware of the complex process that their physician may go through before arriving at a diagnosis and prescribing a treatment. However, anyone involved in medical decision making, or who studies it, can testify that medical decision making is a complex process that requires the physician to apply expert judgment in the face of incomplete information, a process often described as decision making under uncertainty.

Hunink et al. (2011) noted that the number of treatments available in medicine has rapidly expanded in recent years. For instance, the first edition of the *Merck Manual*, a medical reference book first published in 1899, was 192 pages long, whereas the 1999 edition of the *Merck Manual* was 2,833 pages long. Other factors complicating the decision-making process include the fact that many more diseases have been recognized than was the case decades ago. In addition, many treatment options are "halfway" measures that do not cure a condition but improve the patient's health or quality of life, and even if the diagnosis is correct, the outcome of the treatment may be uncertain. Finally, concerns about the costs of different treatments may play a role in the decision-making process, even if they are not directly articulated.

Medical decision making is sometimes studied by applying a body of techniques first developed in the business world to help clarify the decision-making process and allow decision makers to recognize and explicitly include or exclude all relevant information in the process of making their choices. While it is impossible to reduce the process of decision making in medicine to a mathematical formula, the use of explicit procedures may make the process more transparent and reliable and may lead to better decisions.

Hunink et al. (2011) provided examples of several types of decision-making procedures that may be useful to physicians. One is a consequence table, which lists the probable consequences of a particular medical decision on a particular condition. For instance, for the common childhood condition of "glue ear" (i.e., otitis media with effusion), they list the consequences of the "wait-and-see" approach (doing nothing initially, to see if the condition will resolve without treatment) with regard to hearing, behavior, language development, acute middle ear infection, and long-term complications. Similar tables could be constructed for other treatment options, and having the consequences stated explicitly can facilitate comparison and thus aid in choosing which treatment to follow.

Another potentially useful tool in medical decision making is the decision tree. In this technique, the options for treatment and their possible consequences are written in a tree diagram, with the problem on the left and the treatments and consequences depicted on branches on the right. For instance, if three potential treatments for a sore throat are under consideration, each would get its own "branch" stemming from the condition in question. The potential consequences of each treatment are then listed on separate branches stemming from each potential treatment, often with probabilities attached (for instance, the probability that the choice to employ "watchful waiting" could lead to a more serious infection).

A third tool in medical decision making is the clinical balance sheet. This is a table showing the alternatives for treating a condition and the potential benefits, harms, and costs of each. For instance, Huninck et al. (2011) presented a clinical balance sheet for three options for treating glue ear: monitoring ("wait and see"), short-term insertion of a tube, and use of a hearing aid. For each, the potential treatment benefits are listed in the categories of hearing and behavior, language development, acute infections, and long-term complications, and potential treatment harms and costs are listed in the categories of long-term complications of the treatment, restrictions, short-term complications, and costs. As with the consequence table and decision tree, the clinical balance sheet is not intended to replace expert judgment (in fact, expert judgment is required to create the balance sheet in the first place), but to aid in the decision-making process by clearly stating the choices and their possible outcomes.

PHYSICIAN AND PHARMACIST EDUCATION

The World Health Organization (WHO) issued a list of 10 recommendations for prescribers and dispensers as part of its global strategy to combat antimicrobial resistance. Four of these recommendations were highlighted as priorities: educating prescribers and dispensers (including pharmacists and others who sell drugs) on the importance of appropriate use of antimicrobials and of containing antimicrobial resistance; educating prescribers on issues of disease control and prevention; promoting education at the undergraduate and postgraduate levels in the diagnosis and management of common infections; and encouraging development of treatment guidelines and algorithms.

Six other recommendations were included as lower priorities: encouraging prescribers and dispensers to educate patients about appropriate antibiotic use; educating prescribers and dispensers about factors such as economic incentives and pharmaceutical promotions that may influence their prescribing practices; using supervision and support to improve clinical practices; auditing prescribing and dispensing practices and providing feedback to prescribers; allowing formulary managers to limit antimicrobial use (e.g., requiring a prescription, allowing a selected range of appropriate antimicrobials), and requiring training and continuing education in antimicrobial use as a professional registration requirement for prescribers and dispensers.

Medical School Education

Medical school typically includes classes in topics such as pharmacology and pharmacotherapy. However, some physicians graduate feeling unprepared in the actual practice of prescribing appropriate drugs to their patients, and research has indicated that recently graduated physicians are more likely to make errors in medication than physicians with many years of experience. One proposed reason for this situation is the way that physicians are educated: during clinical training, the emphasis is on symptoms and diagnoses, while pharmacology training focuses on particular drugs and their uses, rather than beginning with patients and finding the best drug (if any) to treat their condition.

In the mid-1990s, a team led by T. P. G. M. de Vries produced the *Guide to Good Prescribing*, which was developed in cooperation with the World Health Organization Action Programme on Essential Drugs and published by the WHO. The *Guide* identified a six-step process for rational prescribing, developed from a model based on an observation study of prescribing practices in the Netherlands. It also was reviewed by experts from 30 countries before publication. While intended for use in medical school, the *Guide* could be used by physicians already practicing who want a model on which to base their own prescribing practices.

The six steps identified in the *Guide* are to define the patient's problem, taking into account both symptoms and probable causes; specify the therapeutic objective; choose an appropriate drug and verify that it will be effective and safe for the specific patient (e.g., some drugs should not be taken during pregnancy; some drugs are not appropriate for a person who drives for a living); begin treatment, including an explanation to the patient of how to take the drug and why it is important; give the patient information about the drug, including any warnings (e.g., to abstain from alcohol while taking it); and monitor the treatment for effectiveness and change or end the treatment if appropriate.

Although the *Guide* covers prescribing practices for all types of medical conditions, it contains a number of examples pointing out common errors in the prescription of antibiotics. These uses are unlikely to help the patient but can lead to the development of antibiotic resistance. One example of inappropriate use of antibiotics is prescribing a broad-spectrum antibiotic when a narrow-spectrum antibiotic would perform as well for the patient. Another inappropriate use is prescribing antibiotics for mild dehydration and watery diarrhea when the focus should be on rehydration and the prevention of further dehydration. A third is the use of antibiotics, either local or systemic, to treat open wounds. Because most wound infections carry little danger of infection, cleaning and dressing the wound constitute the recommended treatment in most cases, together with telling the patient to return for more care if the wound becomes infected. Patient vignettes are included to help physicians apply the steps outlined for the prescribing process and differentiate among cases with similar presenting symptoms.

While the steps in the *Guide* may seem obvious, and in fact may be followed by most practitioners today, there is an argument for teaching these steps explicitly as part of medical school training. Tests of the six-step model with medical students in numerous countries established that those trained in it performed better not only in terms of following rational prescribing practices for the types of examples they were trained on, but also applying their knowledge to other medical conditions. Although originally published in 1994, the *Guide* and its six-step model continue to be used in medical school education today.

Effectiveness of Physician Education

Many different types of physician education have been developed to promote the rational use of antibiotics. Educational strategies may be classified as either passive or active. Passive strategies include the distribution of printed materials to physicians, the distribution of clinical guidelines within a hospital, and continuing medical education conducted by traditional methods such as lectures, seminars, conferences, and educational courses. Active methods include discussion groups, educational outreach (personal visits by health professionals), sequenced education sessions, workshops or conferences outside the provider's usual workplace, and methods combining education and practice or simulated practice such as interactive role playing, problem solving, case solving, and hands-on-training.

Yolisa Nalule (2011) summarized the results of many studies conducted in a variety of countries that looked at prescribing behavior and the effectiveness of different types of physician education. She found that inappropriate prescribing of antibiotics associated with working in a rural setting, having been in practice longer, having less access to current medical information, and not being involved in medical teaching.

Nalule found that physician education is moderately successful in reducing inappropriate antibiotic prescribing, with active methods generally more effective than passive methods. However, no single method of physician education proved consistently best, and passive methods still remain in common use, possibly due to their low cost and ease of implementation. In addition, combinations of active and passive methods have been used and sometimes proved more effective than a single method. For instance, one study found that the combination of interactive meetings and passive meetings produced more change in prescribing practices than either passive or interactive meetings alone.

HEALTH SYSTEM GUIDELINES

There are no specific national guidelines governing the use of antibiotics in medicine in the United States, in part because of the decentralized way that healthcare is delivered in this country. However, some hospital and healthcare systems have published detailed guidelines for antibiotic use. While these guidelines are not intended to override the individual judgment of a physician or intrude into the doctor-patient relationship, they provide a summary of the best and most recent information along with recommendations for treatment in specific instances. These guidelines can influence antibiotic use outside the health system for which they were created since they may be adopted as best practices by other systems and practitioners that do not have the personnel to develop their own guidelines.

To take one example, the Cleveland Clinic, an academic medical center including over 3,000 physicians and scientists, with over 5 million patient visits per year, publishes an annual set of guidelines for antibiotic use. The guidelines are updated each year with the latest available information about available treatments, efficacy, and antibiotic resistance, including emerging patterns of resistance. They also contain reference information about subjects such as the Gram stain patterns of common organisms, a table of lab tests and specimen types, and a table of the mechanism of action of common antibacterial agencies. The purpose of the guidelines is to provide the most cost-effective care to patients so that they receive the drugs that they need but are not prescribed unnecessary drugs, which may lead to opportunistic infections or adverse drug reactions, as well as the growth of antimicrobial resistance.

CHAPTER 8

Changing Patient Behavior

It is a common assumption that if a drug is prescribed to a patient, that patient will take the drug as directed. This assumption incorporates several other assumptions: that the correct drug will be obtained, in the correct dosage, and that it will be taken at appropriate intervals for the appropriate length of time. These assumptions ignore the issue of patient adherence to treatment (the term *adherence* is often preferred to *compliance* because it acknowledges the active role that the patient takes in his or her own treatment), a topic of increasing interest in medical and health research today. Patient adherence is important because it is associated with better patient outcomes, while nonadherence is associated with poorer outcomes and, in the case of nonadherence with antibiotic medications, with the development of resistant strains of microbes.

PATIENT ADHERENCE

Patient adherence is difficult to measure. The most accurate information would be obtained by direct observation of the patient over the entire recommended course of treatment, an ideal that is generally not possible to attain for patients living in the community (as opposed to those who are hospitalized, for instance). Researchers have used a variety of methods, from self-reporting to recording devices installed on pill containers, to gather data about medication adherence, but their accuracy varies. For instance, people often exaggerate their adherence behavior when asked to report on it, while mechanical systems of collecting data are likely to be more accurate. Reported differences in adherence may be due in some cases to differing systems of measurement, making it difficult to determine what factors are most influential in medication adherence.

In addition, there are several different aspects to adherence, and researchers in different studies may use different definitions of what constitutes adherence to a treatment regimen (e.g., must 100 percent of the doses be taken as supplied, or does 80 percent enough to count as adherence?). Many studies assess adherence across several dimensions and may report different levels of adherence for each dimension. Two commonly used definitions of adherences are compliance and persistence. *Compliance* is defined as the percentage of doses taken as prescribed, while *persistence* is defined as the number of days taking a prescribed medication.

The opposite of adherence is nonadherence. There are many ways that a patient can be nonadherent, including not filling the prescription at all, not refilling the prescription as necessary, not picking up the prescription after it has been filled, skipping doses of medication, failing to complete a course of treatment (stopping the medication early), or taking a dosage different than what was prescribed. In the latter case, an individual might take too large a dose, in which case she or he might become ill or run out of the medication too soon, or take too small a dose, in which case the medication might be ineffective. Some researchers have also identified more specific types nonadherence, such as *drug holidays*, when a patient stops taking the medication as prescribed for a period of time and then begins again to take it as prescribed, and *white coat compliance*, when a patient takes medication as prescribed around the time of medical appointments, but not at other times.

Research into Patient Adherence

Most studies have found surprisingly low levels of patient adherence. For instance, among people prescribed long-term medication therapy, adherence rates have often been found to be in the range of 40 to 50 percent (meaning that half or more of patients do not adhere to their prescribed medication regimen). Adherence has been found to be more common in short-term regimens, typically in the range of 70 to 80 percent, but that still leaves 20 to 30 percent of patients not following their medication protocol as prescribed.

Adherence to medication regimens also has been found to vary according to the specific disease treated. For instance, one study found that adherence to prescription drug regimens for asthma was about 50 percent, while adherence to prescription drug regimens for hypertension (high blood pressure) was in the range of 50 to 75 percent. Adherence to oral medication regimes prescribed for Type II diabetes have been found to range from 65 to 85 percent, while adherence to insulin administration regimes has been measured at about 20 percent.

According to the American College of Preventive Medicine (ACPM), in the United States, for every 100 prescriptions written, 50 to 70 go to a pharmacy, and only 48 to 66 are picked up at the pharmacy. Obviously, if a prescription is not filled and picked up, the patient will not be taking the medicine, and about one-third of all prescriptions written in the United States fail at this point in the process. Continuing with the ACPM data, about 25 to 30 percent of prescriptions are taken properly, and 15 to 20 are refilled as prescribed. These figures indicate another reason for varying estimates of adherence in different studies: They depend on when the measurement of adherence begins. If a study begins with the patient already having obtained the correct medicine, then one key factor in nonadherence has been eliminated.

Besides representing a danger both to the health of the individual patient and to public health (the latter due to the development of drug-resistance microbes, as well as the increased presence of contagious disease in a community), medication nonadherence creates a significant economic burden on society. The ACPM estimates that nonadherence imposes an economic burden in the United States of $100 to $300 million annually, in part due to increased admissions to hospitals and nursing homes.

Studies focusing on adherence to antibiotic prescriptions for particular diseases have also found low rates of compliance. For instance, a 2013 study by Llor and colleagues of 428 adult patients with acute lower respiratory tract infections or bacterial pharyngitis used the Mediation Event Monitoring System (MEMS) to monitor patient adherence. MEMS uses a medication bottle with a microelectronic chip that records the date and time when the bottle is opened, with the assumption that opening the bottle means the patient is taking the medication. Because it does not rely on self-reporting, but rather records a behavior logically connected with taking the medicine in question, MEMS is considered a highly accurate way to measure adherence. Llor and colleagues found that only 30 percent of patients achieved excellent adherence, with 12.4 percent showing acceptable adherence, 28.7 percent declining adherence over time, and 28.5 percent unacceptable adherence or nonadherence.

A literature review by Jin et al. (2008) found numerous factors related to medication adherence in various studies, although frequently the results of different studies were contradictory. For instance, some studies have found that older patients (defined specifically for each study, but often defined as those over 55 or 60 years of age) are more adherent than average, while other studies found them to be less adherent. In contrast, many studies have found that young adults (typically defined as those younger than 30 or 40) are less adherent than average, and some studies have found that children and adolescents with chronic diseases are less adherent than the average patient.

Some studies have found that white patients are more likely to be adherent to medication regimens than Black or Hispanic patients, although this result may be confounded by issues such as income, education, and health literacy. There is no clear pattern regarding gender: Some studies found women to be more adherent, some found women less adherent, and some found no difference in adherence between men and women. Similarly, higher educational level in some studies is associated with greater adherence, in others with lower adherence, and in yet others, no difference is found by educational level. One fairly consistent finding, however, is that married people are more adherence than the unmarried—five studies found this result, with none finding the contrary pattern, although five other studies found no difference in adherence between married and unmarried people.

Many other factors have also been studied in relation to medication adherence. Although results are sometimes contradictory, increased number of doses per day, longer duration of treatment, taking multiple medications, and side effects from medication generally are associated with lower adherence, while convenient route of medication administration is associated with increased adherence. Low income and lack of health insurance also have been found to be negatively related to adherence, while social support is positively related to adherence. In addition, poor adherence is related to difficulties with the healthcare system, long waiting times at clinics, poor experiences with medical visits, and difficulties in getting prescriptions filled, while satisfaction with clinic visits is positively associated with adherence.

OBSTACLES TO ADHERENCE

Medication adherence is a complex issue. The World Health Organization (WHO) has identified five dimensions of medication adherence: social and economic factors, healthcare system factors, condition-related factors, therapy-related factors, and patient-related factors.

Examples of social and economic factors that may influence medication adherence include health literacy, insurance, cost of medications, cultural beliefs about illness, and unstable living conditions. Each of these factors may manifest itself in different ways with different patients: for instance, a person lacking in health literacy may be unable to understand the directions provided for taking the medications prescribed, or he or she may not understand or value the reasons given for taking the medication as provided. Similarly, the cost of medication may present a barrier to compliance in many ways—the patient may not fill the prescription at all, may obtain a drug of inferior quality outside the official pharmaceutical channels, or may take a lower dosage than prescribed in order to make the drug last longer.

Healthcare system factors include the quality of the patient-provider relationship, healthcare professionals' knowledge regarding adherence and ways to promote it, continuity of care, required copays for prescription drugs, communication between the provider/system and the patient, and restrictions on available medications due to drug formularies. These factors place some of the responsibility for medication adherence on the healthcare system, rather than considering it solely the personal responsibility of the patient. For instance, professionals within the healthcare system should understand the importance of medication adherence, be aware of ways to promote it, and be able to communicate with patients so that they also understand the importance of adherence. In addition, factors related to health insurance, such as the amount of copayment required to fill a prescription or the restricted availability of certain drugs, also may influence medication adherence.

Condition-related factors include whether the illness being treated is acute or chronic, the type and severity of symptoms, and the presence of mental illness or developmental disability. For instance, a patient may think of a medication in terms of how well it relieves the symptoms of a disease, and if the disease does not manifest obvious symptoms, then he or she may not think that it is important to take the medication. Similarly, a patient may cease taking the medication as prescribed once the symptoms are relieved but before the prescribed course of treatment is completed, a practice that encourages the development of drug-resistant microbes. In addition, if a patient has a mental illness such as depression, or a developmental disability, either may interfere with adherence to medication instructions.

Therapy-related factors include the number of doses of medication prescribed, the method of administration (e.g., oral, injection, by inhaler), the duration of the prescribed therapy, side effects of the medication, immediacy of benefit (i.e., are the patient's symptoms quickly relieved by the drug?) and changes in the prescribed medications or pattern of taking them. If the schedule of medication is complex (for instance, multiple doses of multiple drugs to be taken on a daily basis), that adds to the cognitive burden of medication adherence, as may changes in the medication schedule. Similarly, the route of administration may affect adherence—for instance, an asthma patient may have difficulty using an inhaler correctly and may give up if it does not provide relief. Patient perception of the effectiveness of therapy is another factor in adherence—for instance, if the symptoms of disease are not relieved fairly quickly, the patient may believe that the medication is not effective and thus stop taking it.

Patient-related factors include physical impairments (e.g., difficulties in seeing or hearing), knowledge of the disease and the treatment protocol, perceived benefits of treatment, motivation to comply with treatment, the stigma carried by the disease, and alcohol or substance abuse. Discussions of medication adherence sometimes assume an ideal patient, while real patients may have difficulties with reading the label on a medication bottle, lack a basic understanding of their disease and the treatment protocol, abuse alcohol or other substances, or be unmotivated to comply with treatment. They also may be reluctant to even acknowledge that they have a disease, especially if they feel that it carries a stigma, and thus they may not be inclined to adhere to a treatment regimen.

Of course, multiple factors may be at play with any particular patient: for instance, cost, lack of health literacy, and a poor relationship with the primary healthcare provider may all present barriers to the same patient, and removing one barrier may not be sufficient to move the patient toward medication compliance. In addition, these factors may interact, creating more complex barriers to medication adherence.

INTERVENTIONS TO IMPROVE ADHERENCE

Many studies indicate that simple interventions can do much to improve medication adherence. Agreja et al. (2005) summarized interventions known to improve adherence under the acronym SIMPLE:

- Simplify the regimen.
- Impart knowledge.
- Modify patient beliefs and human behavior.
- Provide communication and trust.
- Leave the bias (i.e., don't discriminate or make assumptions).
- Evaluate adherence.

The ACPM has provided a number of simple scripts that physicians and other healthcare providers may use to promote medication adherence in the 2011 resource *Medication Adherence Clinical Reference.*

Simplify the regimen. Atreja and colleagues note that a complex treatment regimen may affect compliance adversely, and they recommend that treatment regimens be made as simple as possible. For instance, if medication can be taken once a day rather than three or four times per day (assuming that the medication is available in a one-a-day format and the cost is not prohibitive), that makes the regimen simpler to follow. Similarly, if the timing of medication can be tied to a daily routine, such as taking one pill with each meal, compliance may increase. Other ways to simplify a medication regime include customized packaging tied to the way that a patient will take the drug (e.g., all pills for one time of day in one packet), use of adherence aids and reminders, and dividing the medication regime into steps and explaining each step to the patient.

Impart knowledge. While patient education alone may not improve adherence, combining increased patient knowledge with effective communication and a simplified medication regimen may improve compliance. Recommendations included under this action include clear written and verbal instructions presented in simple language and focused on the most important points, shared decision making between provider and patient, inclusion of the patient's family and friends in the educational efforts if appropriate, provision of information through multiple channels, and reiteration of important information.

Modify patient beliefs and human behavior. Atreja and colleagues suggest a number of ways that patients can be encouraged to modify their behavior toward greater medication adherence. One is to encourage patients to take an active role in managing their condition, ask patients what they need and what would help them become adherent, and address their stated barriers to adherence, including any fears that they may have about the medication. Another suggestion is to be sure that they understand the negative consequences of nonadherence. In some situations, contingency contracting and the provision of rewards for adherence may be appropriate. In contingency contracting, an agreement is created that states the goals for the patient's adherence and provides rewards for fulfilling the contract.

Provide communication and trust. Good communication and trust between healthcare providers and patients is an important factor in promoting medication adherence because while the physician may prescribe the medication, it is the patient who must carry out the treatment plan. Numerous studies have found that physicians are often weak in communication skills: for instance, one study found that half of patients leave a physician's office without understanding what the physician wished to communicate to them. Similarly, physicians may have poor listening skills and thus not create a relationship of trust with the patient: one study found that when a patient is describing symptoms, the person is frequently interrupted by the physician. Many methods are available to improve physician-patient communication, including teaching physicians interviewing and active listening skills and training them to provide appropriate emotional support for each patient, as well as clear information about their condition and the treatment regime.

Leave the bias. Many research studies have found that health outcomes are correlated with patient factors such as income, ethnicity, and educational level. However, physicians and other healthcare providers can take a number of measures to address these disparities. These actions include learning about health literacy, addressing potential communication problems such as language or cultural differences, adopting a patient-centered style of communication, and providing educational materials appropriate to each patient (including factors such as primary language and level of education).

Evaluate adherence. Physicians and other healthcare providers need to collect information about medication adherence among their patients constantly. The simplest way to do this is, at each appointment, to ask patients if they are following their prescribed drug protocol and about barriers to adherence. Because self-report information is often biased in favor of social desirability (i.e., the patient may give the response that he or she believes the physician wants to hear—namely, that the patient is compliant—rather than the true answer), other methods can also be used to measure adherence. These include reviewing the dates when prescriptions are filled and refilled, counting the number of remaining pills in the bottle, or measuring the level of the drug in a patient's blood or urine.

CHAPTER 9

Balancing Individual and Societal Rights

The growth of drug-resistant organisms highlights a basic conflict between two ways of looking at health and medical issues: as a personal matter between a patient and that person's healthcare provider, and as a public health issue, which takes into account the impact on other people of choices made at the patient-provider level. Sometimes individual and societal rights conflict: for instance, a patient using antibiotics inappropriately may foster the growth of drug-resistant microbes that may infect other people. Two specific measures that have been developed to balance the needs and rights of individual patients with that of the great society are directly observed therapy (DOT), developed to combat the growth of drug-resistant tuberculosis (TB), and involuntary quarantine, an ancient practice used to prevent the spread of disease.

BALANCING INFECTION CONTROL AND THE RIGHT TO FREEDOM AND PRIVACY

In the United States, we tend to take an individual approach to issues of medicine and healthcare. This means that we think of an individual's illness or health is a matter primarily of that person's own concern, with health decisions made by him or her, in concert with family members and healthcare providers. In addition, we place a high value on the individual right to privacy in matters of health and medicine, so that in most cases, people are entitled to confidentiality in matters such as whether they have been diagnosed with an illness, are receiving treatment, or have been prescribed drugs or other therapies. Similarly, medical providers have been taught to think primarily in terms of what is best for each patient and to safeguard the privacy of that patient unless the patient desires otherwise.

There is another way of looking at health and medical care, in which the focus is on the larger community or society. This is primarily the province of public health, which is concerned with the overall health of a population. The two views are not always in conflict, and many public health measures are already part of the daily existence of many people, so they pass unnoticed. For instance, in many countries, the provision of clean drinking water is assumed to be available without any individual making a specific effort to procure it because government-provided municipal water systems provide clean water to every household.

Most of the time, the individual and public ways of looking at medicine and healthcare coexist peacefully. However, from time to time, the needs or desires of the individual may conflict with the best interests of the population. For instance, if a person has a contagious disease for which there is no effective treatment, should the person be allowed to act in ways that might spread the disease to other people? If parents object to immunization of their children on philosophical grounds, should the children still be allowed to attend public school, even if in so doing they threaten the health of children who cannot be immunized for medical reasons? If many people choose not to immunize their children, so that herd immunity is threatened, does that make a difference? If an individual has a history of failing to complete the prescribed course of antibiotic therapy for a contagious disease, thus creating conditions favoring the creation of antibiotic-resistant microbes that could infect others, how should the medical and legal system respond?

DOT

DOT is a method devised to help patients adhere to a treatment plan by having them take their prescribed medications in the presence of a healthcare worker or other trained individual. DOT was developed in response to the emergence of drug-resistant TB, a problem that was created in part by TB patients failing to complete the prescribed course of treatment, thus creating an environment in their body that favored the development of drug-resistant microbes. Because TB in a contagious disease, the problem of individuals infected with drug-resistant TB was viewed as a problem not only for the infected individual, but also for the community. The fact that new strains of TB did not respond to the usual drugs raised concerns because of the possibility that the drug-resistant strains of TB could spread through a community.

DOT may be provided in a healthcare facility (clinic-based DOT) or in any other setting (field-based DOT). While clinic-based DOT may seem a more obvious way of providing medical treatment, sometimes field-based DOT is preferable because it removes barriers to treatment. Field-based DOT may be provided in any safe location where the patient and healthcare worker agree to meet, including the patient's home or workplace, a school, or a restaurant, or another public place. If field-based DOT is used, particular care must be exercised to ensure that the patient's confidentiality is not violated. DOT may be administered by a responsible individual other than a healthcare worker (e.g., a work supervisor or clergy member), but the Centers for Disease Control and Prevention (CDC) recommends that a family member not be given this responsibility because the relative's strong emotional ties to the patient may cause a conflict of interest if the patient does not comply with treatment.

The CDC has identified four steps in administering a DOT program: check for side effects, verify the medication, watch the patient take the medication, and document the visit. In the first step, the healthcare worker asks patients about any adverse side effects that they may be experiencing and refers the patient to a physician if necessary. In the second step, the healthcare worker confirms that the correct drugs, in the correct amounts, are being delivered to the patient. In the third step, the healthcare worker watches the patient take the medications, which means that the patient is observed continuously, for example, from the time each pill is delivered until each pill is swallowed. If necessary, the healthcare worker may need to ensure that pills are actually swallowed by checking the patient's mouth, and may require the patient to remain in the clinic for half an hour after taking the pills so that they may not be vomited out. In the fourth step, the healthcare worker documents the visit and whether the medication was administered, and creates a follow-up plan if the medication was not administered.

Besides the protocol to be followed for each DOT visit, the CDC specifies other case management aspects that may be included in a DOT program. These include offering incentives to patients who keep appointments, helping patients with other aspects of their lives that may affect their adherence to the DOT schedule (e.g., assistance in finding housing), providing effective patient education, and helping patients keep appointments (e.g., by reimbursing the cost of transportation).

The World Health Organization (WHO) includes DOT as a key aspect of combating TB on a global basis. The WHO recognizes five key components of an effective DOT program: political commitment, including sufficient funding; high-quality bacteriological services to detect TB cases; a standardized system of treatment, including adequate supervision and patient support; a sufficient supply of effective anti-TB drugs and effective management of them; and an appropriate monitoring and evaluation system, including measurement of the impact of DOT programs.

DOT has both advantages and disadvantages, so the decision of whether to require it of a particular individual requires balancing all the relevant factors. The primary advantage of DOT for the patient is that it ensures that they take the correct medication on schedule, thus receiving the most effective treatment for their disease. In addition, patients are monitored for side effects and have a regular opportunity to discuss their treatment with a healthcare worker. The advantages of DOT from a public health point of view include increasing the probability that the patient completes the appropriate treatment for the disease in question, thus becoming noninfectious earlier; avoiding behavior that promotes the creation of drug-resistant bacteria; and providing regular opportunities to monitor patients and attempt to solve any problems that might interfere with their completing the prescribed course of treatment.

However, DOT also has disadvantages, and these must be weighed against its advantages. From the point of view of the health system, DOT is time consuming and labor intensive to administer, so it is expensive, requiring the investment of resources that are then not available to meet other needs. It is also time consuming for patients, and so patients may view it as insulting, demeaning, or punitive, suggesting that they are not sufficiently able or responsible to follow medical instructions on their own.

INVOLUNTARY QUARANTINE

Quarantine is an ancient method of disease control and prevention that long predates scientific understanding of the causes of disease. The term simply means isolating people who are believed to have a disease, or who may be carrying a disease, from the healthy population. The same principle may be applied to animals: for instance, many countries still require pets or other animals brought into a country to be placed in quarantine for a fixed number of days to ensure that they are not carrying any diseases that might infect other animals in the country. Early quarantine procedures often focused on specific diseases, such as those which were particularly dreaded (such as leprosy, also known as Hansen's disease), or which were not endemic to a country but were known to cause widespread death if introduced (such as the bubonic plague, also called the Black Death).

Although the term *quarantine* is not used, the practice of isolating the ill from the healthy is mentioned in the books of Leviticus and Numbers in the Old Testament. For instance, Leviticus 13:46 states that persons with leprosy must live apart from others and are considered unclean so long as they have the disease. Subsequent sections of Leviticus mention specific signs of infection with leprosy and states that clothing that shows signs of leprosy must be isolated or burned. Numbers 5.1 and subsequent sections state that if a person has leprosy or a discharge, they must be expelled from the camp so that they will not "defile" it (translations vary).

Historical records indicate that various types of quarantine were used in different countries, most based either on isolating ill people from the well, restricting the movement of people who arrive from distant lands, or both. For instance, in the year 549, Justinian, emperor of the Byzantine Empire, created a law to isolate and restrict the movement of people arriving from regions where the plague was known to exist. In the 7th century, China placed restrictions on the ability of people arriving from foreign countries to enter the country.

Across Europe, special institutions were created for the isolation and treatment of lepers, with approximately 19,000 in existence by the 13th century. Such institutions were sometimes erected outside city walls, to isolate infected individuals further. Even if no institution was available to treat individuals infected with leprosy, lepers might be required to leave the city. For instance, in the town of Reggio, Italy, a command was issued in 1374 that persons infected with the plague be removed from the city, which meant that they would be left on their own to either recover or die.

One well-known example of institutionalized quarantine procedures, which some historians consider the first example of quarantine in the modern sense, was enacted in the port city of Venice, Italy, in 1348. That year, the ruling council was given the right to detain ships, passengers, and cargo arriving in the city for up to 40 days (that period of time gave rise to the term *quarantine,* from the Italian word for 40, *quaranta.* These measures were instituted in response to epidemics of the bubonic plague, which some experts believe caused the death of one-third of Europe's population. In 1403, Venice created an isolation station on an island in the Venetian lagoon, believed to be the first maritime isolation station in the world.

The reason the quarantine period was set at 40 days is not clear. Some historians believe that it might have been based on the ancient Greek belief that a contagious disease would develop within 40 days after a susceptible person was exposed to it. Another possibility is that the 40-day period was chosen by cities in a largely Christian Europe because periods of 40 days are mentioned in the Bible in association with key events such as the Great Flood, the time Jesus spent in the wilderness, and the time Moses spent on

Mount Sinai; in addition, the period of Lent, which occupied a key place in the Medieval Christian calendar, also lasts 40 days.

Other cities also established quarantine laws, although the length of the quarantine was sometimes set at 30 rather than 40 days. The city of Ragusa, Italy, passed a law in 1377 that imposed restrictions on people who arrived at the city after having been in areas where the plague was endemic. These individuals were required to remain in isolation for one month before being allowed to enter Ragusa, and anyone from Ragusa who entered the isolation area was also required to remain in isolation for one month. Similar laws were introduced in many other Italian cities, including Genoa, Venice, Marseilles, and Pisa.

Quarantine practices continued to be enacted in the 17th and 18th centuries, and in the Western hemisphere as well as the Eastern. For instance, Boston, Massachusetts, passed an ordinance in 1647 requiring ships entering the harbor to stop for inspection. In 1663, New York City passed a law prohibiting people coming from areas where smallpox was active to enter until they had been inspected by city sanitary officials. By the end of the 17th century, all the major cities on the East Coast of the United States had passed quarantine laws, although they were sometimes enforced only when epidemics were perceived as a particular threat.

In 1663, England required ships bound for London to stop for 40 days at the mouth of the Thames River before proceeding, in an effort to keep the plague from entering the city. This was followed in 1712 by the Quarantine Act, passed in response to a plague epidemic in northern Europe, which required a mandatory quarantine of 40 days for ships and prohibited unloading cargo during this period.

Some U.S. cities created offshore locations for quarantine stations to keep them separate, in the hopes of preventing the introduction of disease. In 1738, a quarantine station was created on Bedloe's Island in New York Harbor in response to the threat of smallpox and yellow fever entering the city. In 1799, Philadelphia creates a quarantine station about 10 miles south of the city, on the Delaware River, in response to a yellow fever epidemic.

In the 19th century, quarantine procedures become more official and consistent. For instance, in 1863, the state of New York created a quarantine office staffed by an official who had the power to detain ships or order that their cargo be removed and the ship be cleaned and fumigated. In 1879, the U.S. Congress created the National Board of Health, partly as an attempt to create more effective and consistent quarantine procedures on a national basis; however, this body was not effective and was dissolved in 1883. In 1893, the National Quarantine Act created a national system of quarantine for the United States, with uniform standards for medical inspections of ships, immigrants, and cargo.

While many quarantine laws were focused on people entering a country, some dealt with internal quarantine (i.e., the quarantine of individuals within a country). For instance, the New York City Department of Health created a quarantine facility for TB patients in 1903; one of the most famous residents was Mary Mallon, also known as "Typhoid Mary." Children infected with polio in a 1916 epidemic in New York City were removed from their homes and placed in quarantine, although this law was not enforced uniformly across all income classes.

In 1949, Seattle created a locked ward for TB patients to compel them to accept treatment and to prevent them from spreading the disease to others. This approach was somewhat reflected in a practice adopted in New York City in the 1990s in response to the spread of multidrug-resistant TB (MDR TB), in which people who refuse treatment are confined to a hospital and required to accept treatment.

Air Travel and Quarantine

While many early quarantine laws were directed at passengers, crew, and cargo arriving by ship, the growth of air travel in the 20th and 21st centuries meant that officials needed to consider ways to prevent the introduction and spread of disease through air travel. The most notable example of this may be the response to the Ebola outbreak of 2014.

Ebola, also known as Ebola hemorrhagic fever, is a disease transmitted by a virus that has a case fatality rate of about 50 percent (that is, about half the people who develop Ebola die from it). It has an incubation period of 2 to 21 days, with the phrase *incubation period* designating the time from an individual becoming infected until he or she begins to show symptoms. Asymptomatic individuals are not infectious. The early symptoms of Ebola, including fever, headache, sore throat, and muscle pain, are shared with many other diseases, making diagnosis difficult.

The 2014 Ebola outbreak began in West Africa, eventually affecting multiple countries, including Guinea, Liberia, and Sierra Leone. Because healthcare delivery is challenging in these countries, many healthcare professionals from Western countries volunteered to help treat Ebola patients in West Africa. In treating patients, they ran the risk of contracting the disease (which is spread through contact with blood and other bodily secretions of infected people), so some Western countries imposed quarantine requirements on individuals who had contact with Ebola patients or traveled in regions where Ebola was active.

For instance, the CDC issued guidelines in 2014 requesting airline crews to screen passengers. This screening involved asking passengers if they had visited Guinea, Liberia, or Sierra Leone in the prior 21 days, and if so, if they had symptoms associated with Ebola, including fever, severe headache, muscle pain, vomiting, diarrhea, stomach pain, or unexpected bleeding or bruising. Due to prior regulations, airline crews were allowed to deny boarding to passengers with serious contagious diseases, and they also were asked to apply this judgment to people who might be infected with Ebola. If a person became ill on a flight, the CDC instructed crew members to assess the Ebola risk by asking the person if they had been exposed to the disease, and to observe if symptoms of it were present. In any case, universal precautions, including treating all body fluids as infectious, were recommended for any cases of in-flight illness.

Some U.S. states, including New Jersey, New York, California, and Florida, passed additional regulations intended to prevent persons infected with Ebola from entering the country and to restrict the movements of people who might be infected but did not have symptoms. While the desire to prevent this deadly disease, which was then unknown in the United States, was understandable, the very general nature of the early symptoms of infection raised issues about whether the right of individuals to travel freely was threatened. In addition, some public health officials feared that severe quarantine periods applied to people at minimal risk of spreading the disease could discourage American healthcare workers from lending their assistance to individuals in West Africa.

The most-publicized case involving Ebola, air travel, and involuntary quarantine is probably that of Kaci Hickox, an American nurse who treated Ebola patients in Sierra Leone in 2014 in conjunction with Doctors Without Borders (*Médecins sans Frontières,* or *MSF*). Upon returning to the United States, Hickox was involuntarily quarantined for three days in an isolation tent in New Jersey because she had a low-grade fever and had been working with Ebola patients.

At the time, Hickox challenged her quarantine, saying that a person may register a fever for many reasons, including emotional upset, particularly when the temperature is taken using a no-touch thermometer (which actually measures skin temperature and then converts that reading to estimate internal body temperature). Hickox stated that she was in fact stressed, exhausted, and jet-lagged after an emotionally taxing month of work followed by a long plane flight; and she was annoyed at the unexpected demands placed on her when reentering the United States. She also pointed out that she had adhered to strict infection control procedures while working in Sierra Leone and had shown no fever or other symptoms of Ebola, apart from a single temperature reading at the airport. After being held for several days, Hickox was allowed to leave New Jersey and return to Maine, where she was ordered to observe a form of "home quarantine" whose provisions included not going to work, avoiding public gatherings, and maintaining a distance of at least three feet from other people.

Hickox's case prompted much public discussion about the conflict between the rights of individuals to travel freely and be free from unnecessary restrictions on their liberty and the right of the public to be protected from disease. New Jersey governor Chris Christie stated that with a deadly disease like Ebola, regulations should err on the side of public health, thus justifying the quarantine of individuals who might be infectious while recognizing that some noninfectious individuals also would be quarantined. He also stated that the threat to public health was too great in this case to allow individuals to substitute voluntary self-monitoring for oversight by the state. Public opinion polls conducted at the time indicated that most residents of New Jersey agreed with him.

After her release, Hickox continued to believe that her quarantine was unjust, so she filed a lawsuit against Christie and other state officials, charging them with, among other things, false imprisonment, violation of due process, and invasion of privacy. Her lawsuit also released details of her treatment in the New Jersey airport, including the fact that her initial temperature reading was normal, and that she felt she was treated like a criminal or terrorist, beginning with her initial contact with immigration officials. She also detailed aspects of her treatment that she felt raised her quarantine above the level of a mere "inconvenience," as it was characterized by some public officials, including the fact that she had no knowledge of how long her quarantine would last or what procedures were being used to determine whether she should be allowed to leave or not, that she was not allowed to contact legal counsel for more than a day, for that she was held in a cold, unfurnished room, and that she was not allowed to take a shower or provided with adequate clean clothing. As of September 2016, Hickox's lawsuit against Christie, based on her involuntary detention, was still proceeding through the state court system.

CHAPTER 10

Contributions of Research to the Fight Against Drug Resistance

The antibiotic revolution was facilitated by the discovery of many new classes of antibiotics in the 1940s and 1950s, which both offered treatments for diseases previously not susceptible to existing drugs and gave physicians alternatives for treating diseases caused by organisms that had become resistant to formerly effective drugs. However, the pace of discovery for new antibiotic drugs has slowed over the past half-century, and relatively few new antibiotics are currently undergoing the drug approval process. One way that research can aid in the fight against drug resistance is by encouraging the development of new antibiotics, an effort that can be furthered by financial incentives and international cooperation.

THE DRUG DEVELOPMENT PROCESS

The drug development process is time consuming and expensive. This means that when a new health threat is identified, it may be years before an effective drug to treat it can be developed (and, of course, there is no guarantee that such a drug will even be found at all). It also means that pharmaceutical manufacturers tend to invest their resources in researching drugs that they believe will bring them the greatest financial returns. One result of these financial calculations is that often, more resources are devoted to developing drugs to treat chronic conditions common in developed countries than to developing drugs to treat infectious diseases more common in developing nations.

Because the time to develop new drugs is measured in years, people often speak of new drugs as being "in the pipeline," meaning that they are at some stage in the drug development process. While different countries have different procedures governing drug development, the process required by the U.S. Food and Drug Administration (FDA) is similar to that employed in many industrialized countries. The FDA drug development process involves five stages: (1) discovery and development; (2) preclinical research; (3) clinical research; (4) FDA review; and (5) FDA postmarket safety monitoring.

The *discovery and development* stage involves identifying a promising compound for further development. This process can begin in many ways: for instance, a researcher may note the unanticipated effects produced by an existing drug. The drug discovery process may begin with a researcher observing that an existing treatment produces such effects and deciding to see if those effects can be harnessed for therapeutic purposes. New insights from research may allow the researcher to design a drug specifically to attack one disease or symptom, or new technologies may facilitate the development of different ways of treating a disease. Or a team of researchers may screen thousands of molecular compounds against many different diseases to identify any compounds that may yield beneficial drugs. Most compounds studied in this phase are eliminated early in the process, while those that remain are scheduled for future testing. In the development half of this stage, researchers gather information through experimentation in order to learn how the compound is processed by the body, what side effects are associated with its use, the best way to administer the drug (e.g., orally or by injection), how it compares with other drugs, and its mechanism of action (that is, how the compound achieves its pharmaceutical effect).

In the *preclinical research* stage, two types of research are conducted: *in vitro*, meaning outside a living organism (*in vitro* means "in glass" and refers to lab glassware such as test tubes and petri dishes), and *in vivo*, meaning "in living organisms" (including animals and plants). Preclinical studies are not usually large, but they are designed to provide detailed information on matters such as toxicity levels and dosing. The results of the preclinical stage are used to determine which drugs should be advanced to the next stage: clinical research.

In the *clinical research* stage, drugs are tested in the human body through a series of clinical trials. Because human beings are involved, this phase is highly regulated and has four phases, each of which includes trials conducted to gather specific information and answer particular questions about the compound. In Phase 1, which typically lasts several months, the drug is tested on 20 to 100 volunteers, who may be well individuals or people with the disease that the drug is intended to treat. The purpose of Phase 1 trials is to establish the safety and dosage of the drug, and about 70 percent of new drugs move through this stage successfully. In Phase 2, which typically lasts from several months to two years, the drug is tested on up to several hundred people who have the disease or condition that the drug is intended to treat. The purpose of Phase 2 testing is to determine the drug's efficacy and side effects, and about one-third of drugs pass through this stage successfully.

Many more volunteer research subjects, typically from 300 to 3,000, are involved in Phase 3 trials. These volunteers are people who have the disease or condition that the drug is intended to treat, and the purpose of this phase is to further establish the drug's efficacy and monitor for adverse reactions. Phase 3 typically lasts from one to four years, and 25 to 30 percent of drugs move through this phase successfully. In Phase 4, the drug is tested on several thousand people who have the disease or condition that the drug is intended to treat. The purpose of this phase is to further study the drug's safety and efficacy. Phase 4 testing is conducted with already-approved drugs and is sometimes referred to as "postmarketing" monitoring. Only rarely is a drug removed from the marketplace in this phase.

The fourth stage in the drug approval process, *FDA review*, requires the drug developer to submit a New Drug Application (NDA) to the FDA. The NDA contains detailed information about the drug gathered from all studies and analyses conducted from the preclinical phase through Phase 3 of the clinical research stage. The drug developer also must include the data from studies conducted both within and outside the United States, safety updates, patient information, proposed labeling and directions for use, and information about the research process's compliance with institutional review board procedures.

The NDA is reviewed by a team at the FDA, who must complete their task within 6 to 10 months. The review team is made of up individuals with particular specialties, each of whom reviews the section relevant to his or her technical knowledge; for instance, a medical officer will review the clinical data, while a pharmacologist will review the animal data. In addition, FDA inspectors travel to the clinical study sites and conduct an inspection intended to reveal anything suspicious about the data submitted, such as if some data were fabricated, withheld, or manipulated. When the review is complete, an "action package" is assembled containing the individual reviews, the inspection report, and other relevant information; this action package becomes the official record of the FDA review. The review team also will issue a recommendation on the drug, and a senior FDA official will make the final decision as to whether it should be approved.

If the FDA determines that a drug is safe and effective for its intended use, the drug is approved, and the organization then works with the drug developer on the labeling process, which includes developing and refining prescribing information. If the FDA determines that additional information is required before the drug can be approved, they may require the developer to conduct additional studies (a decision that that developer may appeal).

The fifth stage of the drug approval process, *FDA postmarket safety monitoring*, takes place after the drug has been approved for human use. This stage is necessary because although the previous stages may have involved thousands of human research subjects, this still provides an incomplete picture of the drug's effects on people. For instance, persons approved to take part in clinical trials are often selected in ways (such as age limitations or lack of complicating conditions) that do not make them representative of the entire population of people who may take the drug. Another factor is that some drugs may be taken for many years, and complications that did not occur during the studies conducted as part of the drug approval process may show up when the drug is taken over a longer period of time.

Several mechanisms exist to facilitate reporting problems with drugs that have received FDA approval, including the Internet-based program MedWatch. MedWatch is a searchable database of clinically important safety information about medical products. It includes a portal for individuals to report problems with specific human medical products (including prescription and over-the-counter drugs, dietary supplements, and medical devices); compilations of safety alerts for human medical products; and information about drug safety labeling changes. The FDA is also developing a system of active surveillance, the Sentinel Initiative, to monitor large databases such as electronic health records systems and medical claims databases in order to identify problems with approved drugs. A drug that has been approved by the FDA may be removed from the market later if postapproval surveillance indicates that the risks of the drug outweigh its benefits. Drugs are typically removed from the market for safety reasons, such as the emergence of serious side effects, but evidence about this harm must be balanced by harms that could be caused by withdrawing the drug, particularly if it is the only drug available to treat a serious medical disease or condition. Examples of drugs removed from the market following FDA approval include rofecoxib (Vioxx), diethylstilbestrol (DES), and temafloxacin (Omniflox).

During the FDA postmarket safety monitoring phase, the FDA may continue to conduct inspections of plants (including overseas plants) where the drug is manufactured in order to determine if good manufacturing practices are being followed. If a manufacturer wants to make changes in the original NDA, such as changes to the formulation, dosage, or labeling of the drug, it must file a supplemental application with the FDA.

ANTIBIOTICS IN THE DRUG DEVELOPMENT PIPELINE

As more microorganisms become resistant to existing antibiotics, new drugs must be developed to replace drugs that have become ineffective. Because of the lengthy process required to bring a new drug to market, public health officials monitor what new antibiotics are currently in development. Many people working in medicine and public health have reported their anxiety about the low number of new antibiotics currently in the pipeline, particularly given that the process of microorganisms becoming antibiotic resistant is likely to continue.

Several reasons have been offered for the dearth of new antibiotics in the drug development pipeline. One is that it becomes more and more difficult to come up with novel and effective compounds. Another reason is that pharmaceutical companies, which seek to earn a profit on their products, see antibiotic development as less lucrative than developing other types of drugs. Antibiotics are usually taken for only a short period of time (e.g., 10 days), while drugs to treat chronic conditions such as high blood pressure or diabetes may be taken for years—proving to be far more lucrative. In addition, the greatest health threats in industrialized countries are mostly chronic conditions, and those suffering from these diseases are the customers willing and able to pay high prices for drugs, and over their entire lifetimes. Also, some diseases that have become resistant to one or more existing drugs, such as malaria, are primarily a problem in the developing world, while drug manufacturers are headquartered in countries in the industrialized world.

A survey of major international pharmaceutical companies in 2008 found that only five—AstraZeneca, GlaxoSmithKline, Merck, Novartis, and Pfizer—had active programs to discover new antibiotics. A study that included many smaller firms, also conducted in 2008, found that only 15 of the 167 antibiotics under development had a new mechanism of action, a characteristic that could make them more likely to be effective in treating diseases caused by organisms that are already resistant to one or more existing antibiotics. Most of the 15 drugs in question were in the early stages of development, meaning that it could be years before they are brought to market, if they even make it that far.

On the positive side, scientists know that there are many possible compounds that could create effective antibiotics. For instance, some estimate that less than 1 percent of the bacteria on Earth have been cultured, and many antibiotics were discovered as a by-product of culturing bacteria. This suggests that the problem of new antibiotic development will require a considerable investment of resources if it is to succeed. Some have proposed public-private partnerships to spur the development of new antibiotics, while others have suggested that further international cooperation is the key to the process.

A survey of U.S. drug manufacturers found that as of March 2015, only 36 new antibiotics intended to treat bacterial infections were currently in the clinical stage of the FDA approval process, with an additional 5 antibiotics approved between May 2014 and February 2015. The most frequently approved drug was Avycaz, approved on February 25, 2015. This is a combination of ceftazidime, a cephalosporin, plus avibactam, a novel beta-lactamase inhibitor brought to market by AstraZeneca/Actavis; it is intended to treat complicated infections of the urinary tract and abdomen and and acute kidney infections.

Four antibiotics were approved in 2014. Sivextro (tedizolid phosphate), brought to market by Cubist Pharmaceuticals (a wholly owned subsidiary of Merck), is in the oxazolidinone class and is intended to treat acute bacterial skin and skin structure infections. Dalvance (dalbavancin), brought to market by Actavis, is in the lipoglycopeptide class and is intended to treat acute bacterial skin and skin structure infections. Orbactiv (oritavancin), brought to market by The Medicines Company, is in the glycopeptide class and is intended to treat acute bacterial skin and skin structure infections caused by Gram-positive bacteria, including methicillin-resistant *Staphylococcus aureus* (MRSA). Zerbaxa (ceftazidime plus tazobactam), brought to market by Cubist Pharmaceuticals, is the combination of a novel cephalosporin plus a beta-lactamase inhibitor and is intended to treat complicated urinary tract infections (UTIs), complicated intra-abdominal infections, and acute kidney infection.

Of the 36 antibiotics identified as being in the U.S. pipeline as of March 2015, 8 were in Phase 3, 20 were in Phase 2, and 8 were in Phase 1. The conditions targeted by drugs in Phase 3 (which are the closest to being approved among the drugs still in the approval process) include *Clostridium difficile*–associated diarrhea, bacterial pneumonia, gonorrhea, complicated UTIs, complicated intra-abdominal infections, hospital-acquired bacterial pneumonia, acute bacterial skin and skin structure infections, and prosthetic joint infections.

CHAPTER 11

Antibiotics in Animal Husbandry

There are three primary uses of antibiotics in animal husbandry. The first is therapeutic, meaning that antibiotics are used to treat a specific disease in an ill animal. This type of antibiotic use is generally uncontroversial, usually involving high doses for a limited period of time. The second common type of use is prophylactic, meaning that animals are given low doses of antibiotics over a longer period of time (several weeks or more), usually in their food or drinking water, although they are not ill. This is somewhat more controversial because it involves the administration of large quantities of drugs (although each individual dose is small, widespread administration adds up to large quantities of antibiotics consumed) and large numbers of animals being given antibiotics; in addition, administering low dosages of antibiotics can create the ideal conditions for breeding antibiotic-resistance microorganisms.

The line between therapeutic and prophylactic use is not always clear: for instance, if some animals in a herd become infected with a disease, they will be treated (therapeutic use), but other animals in the herd may also be treated so that they do not become infected (prophylactic use). However prophylactic use in response to an existing infection within a herd can be differentiated from general prophylactic use before any infection is present; the latter type of use is common when animals are raised in crowded conditions that foster disease transmission.

The third common use of antibiotics is for growth promotion, in which case very low doses of antibiotics are given to animals in their feed to increase their growth, productivity, or both. This type of antibiotic use has been banned in many countries (although it is still widespread in the United

States) because it is not necessary for the well-being of the animals and promotes antibiotic resistance.

When used as growth promoters, low doses of antibiotics are included in animal feed on a regular basis, a practice that has been shown to promote more rapid growth and sometimes also a higher-quality product (e.g., meat with a higher protein content). Although the exact means by which antibiotic growth promoters produce these results are unclear, one theory is that the antibiotics change the bacterial population in the intestines of feed animals and decrease the energy lost to microbial fermentation within the intestines, allowing that energy to be used for increased animal growth. Faster growth can result in greater profits for the owner of the herd because feed animals are typically sold based on their weight.

The prophylactic use of antibiotics may be used to prevent disease from spreading through a herd, and to control the growth of pathogens such as *Escherichia coli*, *Salmonella*, *Campylobacter*, and *Enterococci*, which can be transmitted to humans consuming infected meat. Prophylactic use of antibiotics may be used in part to mask the effects of unsanitary practices in animal husbandry by reducing the pathogen load in animals raised in unhygienic conditions. Both the use of antibiotics as growth promoters and the prophylactic use provide advantages to the owner of the herd, but both practices are a public health concern because they promote the development of antibiotic-resistant microbes, some of which pose a threat to humans.

The use of antibiotics as food animal growth promoters differs widely across countries. As stated previously, it is widespread in the United States, while in the European Union, it was prohibited in 2006. In some countries, the prohibition of antibiotic growth promoters dates back even further: in Sweden, for instance, their use was banned in the mid-1980s. While some meat and dairy producers may elect to not use antibiotic growth promoters, even if they are permitted, this decision places the producer at a competitive disadvantage unless he or she is producing for a specific market that is willing to pay higher prices for meat or milk that is certified as being raised without the use of antibiotics.

Although several concerns have been raised about the widespread, nontherapeutic use of antibiotics in animal husbandry (i.e., the use of antibiotics for reasons other than to treat a specific disease affecting a specific animal), the chief one is that this practice promotes the selection of antibiotic-resistant strains of pathogens that may infect humans. The possibility of creating drug-resistant strains of pathogens through the use of antibiotics in animal feed, as well as the transfer of drug-resistant bacteria from animals to humans, have been known since at least the 1970s. For instance, Levy et al. (1976) reported the results of a study at the Tufts University School of Medicine that found that when chickens consumed feed containing low doses of the antibiotic oxytetracycline, strains of *E. coli* resistant to this drug soon appeared in their fecal matter. In addition, drug-resistant strains of *E. coli* were isolated in the fecal matter of people living nearby, although those individuals had not been consuming oxytetracycline.

A similar pattern of results was found in a series of studies conducted in the 1980s in Germany and the Netherlands, which found that antibiotic-resistant streptococcal pathogens could be transmitted from farm animals to humans. These results, as well as those of other research, have established three key principles regarding the use of antibiotics in animal feed: the nontherapeutic use of low doses of antibiotics in animal feed promotes the selection of bacteria resistant to those antibiotics; the same mechanism is responsible for the creation of drug resistance in animals and humans; and the genes for drug resistance can be transmitted from animals to humans through the food chain.

HISTORY

The first studies identifying the growth-promoting effects of antibiotics were conducted in the 1940s. In this research, animals whose feed included residues of chlortetracycline showed improved growth, which was later demonstrated to be due to the way that the antibiotic reacted with the microbes in the animals' intestines. In 1951, the U.S. Food and Drug Administration (FDA) approved the use of antibiotics, without prescription, in animal feed, and in the 1950s and 1960s, many European countries also began allowing their use in animal feed. The adoption of intensive animal husbandry practices, also called *factory farming* (e.g., keeping animals penned at a greater density than would normally be the case), also increased the use of antibiotics. Intensive animal husbandry increases the efficiency by which animal feed was converted into meat and other food products, but it also creates the ideal conditions for the spread of disease among the animals and provides a particular incentive for producers to adopt the routine use of antibiotics.

In 1969, the Swann Committee in the United Kingdom recommended dividing antimicrobial products used in animal husbandry into two classes: those used for therapeutic purposes, with a veterinary prescription, and those used as food additives, without a prescription. This committee also recommended restricting the use of antibiotics as growth promoters. In 1970, the European Economic Community (the EEC, a precursor to the European Union) began harmonizing regulations in member countries regarding the use of antibiotics in animal feed. One result was the establishment of the basic principle that only additives specified by a directive of the EEC could be used in animal feed.

In the early 1970s, the use of tetracycline, penicillin, and streptomycin as feed additives was banned in several countries in Europe. In 1986, Sweden became the first country in the world to ban the use of all antibiotics as growth promoters in animal feed. Although no other country immediately followed with so extensive a ban, many European countries did prohibit the use of certain antibiotics as growth promoters. For instance, avoparcin was banned in Denmark in 1995 and Germany in 1996, and this ban was extended to the entire European Union in 1997.

At a World Health Organization (WHO) meeting in Berlin in 1997, a report called "The Medical Impact of the Use of Antibiotics in Food Animals" recommended halting the use of medically important antibiotics as growth promoters. In 1998, the Copenhagen Recommendations called attention to the threat of antimicrobial resistance and called for the development of a surveillance system in Europe to track the growth of antimicrobial resistance. The same year, Denmark banned the use of virginiamycin as a growth promoter, and Finland banned spiramycin in 1998 as a growth promoter. In 1999, the Scientific Steering Committee of the European Commission recommended phasing out the use of antibiotic growth promoters, and in 2006, all antibiotic growth promoters were banned in the European Union.

SPECIFIC THREATS

While many types of bacteria may be affected by the use of antibiotic growth promoters in animal feed, four are of particular concern because of the threat they pose to human health: *Salmonella*, *Campylobacter*, *E. coli*, and *Enterococci*.

Salmonella bacteria can cause many human diseases, including typhoid fever (caused by *Salmonella typhi*), which can be fatal. However, because typhoid is spread exclusively from one human to another (through fecal contamination of food or water), the use of antibiotics in animal husbandry does not affect this disease in humans. However, other strains of *Salmonella*, including varieties of *Salmonella enterica*, can be transmitted between animals and humans and cause disease in humans. These strains of *Salmonella* most often cause gastroenteritis, with symptoms that may include mild or severe diarrhea, vomiting, and fever, although they also can cause invasive disease that may result in death. Originally, human disease caused by *Salmonella* infection could be treated with several different types of antibiotics, including ampicillin, fluoroquines, and chloramphenicol. However, human cases of food poisoning following consumption of meat or milk containing *Salmonella* strains resistant to at least one of these classes of drugs have been reported in the United States since the 1980s, and resistant strains have since been identified in the United Kingdom and other countries.

Campylobacter species, particularly *Campylobacter coli* and *Campylobacter jejuni*, are common causes of food poisoning in humans. Infection with *Campylocbacter* can cause mild to severe diarrhea, fever, and vomiting, and in rare cases (generally among the very young or very old) may lead to hospitalization or even death. *Campylobacter* species are sensitive to a number of types of antibiotics, and erythromycin, a macrolide, is a common choice of treatment. Because erythromycin is commonly used as a food additive for pigs in the United States, the possible emergence of strains of *Campylobacter* resistant to this antibiotic is a public health concern. *Campylobacter* strains resistant to fluoroquinolones, another antibiotic to which the bacteria was formerly susceptible, have been identified in many countries and have been traced to the use of fluoroquinolones in poultry production.

E. coli is a type of bacteria ordinarily present in the digestive tract of humans and many other types of animals. However, some strains of *E. coli* can cause disease in humans, including urinary tract infections (UTIs), bloodstream infections, and diarrhea. Some strains of *E. coli* are particularly deadly: for instance, infection with *Vero-Toxigenic Escherichia coli* (*VTEC*, also called *E. coli* O157) may lead to renal failure, particularly in children. Antibiotic-resistant strains of *E. coli* have been identified in many countries, and this bacteria seems to be particularly adept at creating resistant strains through horizontal gene transfer.

Enterococci are a type of bacteria associated with many different types of disease, including endocarditis, meningitis, UTIs, and bloodstream infections (bacteremia). Because *Enterococci* are Gram-negative bacteria, they are naturally susceptible to many types of antibiotics, including many commonly used as growth promoters. The use of antibiotics in animal food is suspected as a cause of the development of strains of *Enterococci* that are resistant to multiple types of antibiotics. Drug-resistant strains of *Enterococci* were found in Europe beginning in the 1980s, but now they are also seen in other countries. The use of the antibiotic avoparcin in animal feed is of particular concern because, although avoparcin is not used in human medicine, it is closely related to two antibiotics that are: vancomycin and teicoplanin.

THE SCOPE OF THE ISSUE

In the United States, 70 percent of antibiotics used are consumed by animals, while only 30 percent are consumed by humans. There are no precise statistics on how common antibiotic use is in agriculture around the world, and statistics are not always kept separately for animal husbandry and other agricultural purposes. However, antibiotic use in agriculture other than for animal husbandry is rare (some estimate that 99.6 to 99.8 percent of all agriculture use of antibiotics is for animal husbandry).

While the exact amount of antibiotics used worldwide in agriculture is unknown, it is clear that the use of antibiotics in animal husbandry is common and on at least a scale similar to the use of antibiotics to treat people. Although many countries do not keep data that would allow the precise determination of the quantity of antibiotics used for agricultural purposes, current estimates of the amount of antibiotics used annually in agriculture range from 63,000 tons to almost four times that. Some sources estimate that global use of antibiotics in agriculture will increase by 67 percent between 2010 and 2030. Most (i.e., over 70 percent) of the antibiotics considered important in human use are also used in agriculture, so the development of organisms resistant to these antibiotics has implications for human as well as animal health.

United States

In 2013, 17 classes of drugs were approved for use with food-producing animals in the United States. Tetracyclines were the most commonly used type of antibiotic (44 percent), followed by ionophores (30 percent), and penicillins (6 percent). Both tetracyclines and penicillins are classified by the FDA as medically important for use with humans, while ionophores are not. Among the medically important antibiotics, most were administered through feed (74 percent) or water (21 percent), with the remainder administered by injection (4 percent), orally (1 percent) or intramammary administration (less than 1 percent).

Between 2009 and 2013, the use of medically important antibiotics for food-producing animals increased by 20 percent, from 7.7 million kilograms in 2009 to 9.2 million kilograms in 2013. Over the same period, the use of antibiotics classified as not currently medically important drugs increased by 14 percent, from 4.9 million kilograms to 5.6 million kilograms.

The greatest percentage increase was seen in lincosamides, a medically important drug: an increase of 153 percent, from 0.09 million kilograms to 0.24 million kilograms. The greatest decrease was seen in sulfa drugs, which also are medically important: a decrease of 24 percent, from 0.5 million kilograms to 0.38 million kilograms.

Among medically important drugs, 28 percent were used only for therapeutic indications, while 72 percent were used for production (e.g., increased rate of weight gain) or both production and therapeutic indications (prophylactic use is not reported as a separate category). Among drugs classified as not medically important, 30 percent were used for therapeutic indications only, 1 percent for production indications only, and 69 percent for both production and therapeutic indications.

Europe

The scope of antibiotic use in animal husbandry varies widely from one country to another. For instance, a 2015 study of 26 countries in the European Union (EU) or European Economic Area (EEA) looked at veterinary antibiotic use for food-producing animals using 2013 data. This survey, which covered 95% of the animals used to produce food in the EU/EEA, found wide differences in antibiotic use between countries. Across all 26 countries, the most common antibiotic used for food-producing animals were tetracyclines (36.7% of the total), followed by penicillins (24.5 percent) and sulfonamides (9.6 percent).

In order to facilitate comparison between countries of different sizes, the unit of comparison was veterinary antibiotics sold in the country, expressed in milligrams (mg), per population correction unit (PCU) in kilograms (kg), the latter being a proxy for the size of the animal population in the country. Many things could explain these observed differences in antibiotic use, including policy differences and different compositions of the food animal populations in each country (e.g., some countries might raise relatively more pigs, others relatively more cattle). In 2013, the highest rate of antibiotic use for food-producing animals was found in Cyprus (426 mg/PCU), followed Spain (317 mg/PCU), Italy (302 mg/PCU), and Hungary (230 mg/PCU). The lowest rates were found in Norway (3.7 mg/PCU), Iceland (5.3 mg/PCU), Sweden (13 mg/PCU) and Slovenia (22 mg/PCU).

Overall, a decline of 7.9 percent in antibiotic use for food-producing animals was observed from 2011 to 2013 (data was available over that period for only 23 countries). However, patterns of increase or decrease varied among countries, with 11 countries showing a decrease of more than 5 percent, and 6 showing an increase of more than 5 percent.

Some European countries have adopted policies intended to reduce anti-biotic use in agriculture (most agricultural antibiotics are used on live-stock). For instance, in 1995, Denmark established a surveillance system to monitor antibiotic resistance. The country, which is a major pork exporter, also began a series of steps to ban antibiotic growth promoters in hog pro-duction. This program was successful, as antibiotic use in hog production declined by 51 percent between 1992 and 2008 even though overall hog pro-duction increased by 47 percent over the same period. Over the same period, antimicrobial use in the poultry industry also decreased by 90 percent, while poultry production slightly increased. This example demonstrates that meat production can thrive even while producers decrease or eliminate nontherapeutic antibiotic use.

Drug-Resistant Organisms in Meat

Recognizing the role that antibiotic use in agricultural can play in human health, in 1996, the National Antimicrobial Resistance Monitoring System (NARMS) was created in the United States to protect and promote public health by providing information about drug-resistant organisms, infections caused by them, and the impact of interventions to contain the spread of such organisms.

NARMS studies have found a wide presence of *Salmonella*, including drug-resistant *Salmonella*, in different types of meat available for retail sale. This is concerning not only because it demonstrated how widespread drug-resistant *Salmonella* has become in meat production, but also because people can be infected with *Salmonella* through eating contaminated meat. Following safe handling and cooking procedures (e.g., washing hands and all surfaces used for meat preparation immediately after use, cooking meat at a temperature high enough to kill microorganisms) can reduce the risk, but unexpected events (e.g., a package of meat leaking and contaminating another food) and ordinary human error (e.g., not checking the internal tem-perature of cooked meat before eating it) can occur, such that food con-taminated with bacteria often does cause human illness. We don't know exactly how many cases of food poisoning occur each year because most cases are mild and do not require medical care, but some cases do bring about serious illness or death. In addition, the rise of antibiotic-resistance microorganisms makes the problem of contaminated food more serious.

NARMS studies have found wide variation in the percentage of infected samples depending on the type of meat and the location where the meat was sold. In addition, the specific drugs to which the drug-resistant *Salmo-nella* was resistant showed significant variability. Both types of informa-tion are useful because they can be used to target resources where they are most needed and to identify practices in the regions where contamination is most common that may be leading to the contamination. For instance, a 2013 study of meat sold in retail locations in 14 states (6,646 total packages tested) found that overall, 5.3 percent were contaminated with *Salmonella*. Breaking it down by type of meat, NARMS found that 12.5 percent of the samples of chicken, 6.4 percent of ground turkey, 1.4 percent of pork chops, and 0.9 percent of ground beef were contaminated by *Salmonella*.

The percentage of resistant bacteria among the *Salmonella* isolates found in a specific type of meat was highest in turkey, with 77.4 percent of isolates found to be resistant to at least one antibiotic, and 39.6 percent resistant to at least three classes of antibiotics. Of the *Salmonella* isolates found in chicken, 59.6 percent showed resistance to at least one type of antibiotic, and 26.0 percent were resistant to at least three classes of antibiotics. Among ground beef samples, 53.3 percent of *Salmonella* isolates were found to be resistant to at least one type of antibiotic, and 33.3 percent were resistant to at least three classes of antibiotics. Among pork chop samples, 45.8 percent of *Salmonella* isolates were found to be resistant to at least one antibiotic, with 33.3 percent resistant to at least three classes of antibiotics.

BALANCING PRODUCTIVITY AND PUBLIC SAFETY

The primary concern in animal husbandry is not the use of antibiotics to treat specific diseases in ill animals, but their use to promote growth in healthy animals. Individual meat producers have an incentive to use antibiotics in this way because it helps their livestock gain weight faster, thus shortening the time that it takes to bring animals to market, producing larger or more productive animals, or both, all of which increase profit for the producers. A meat producer who voluntarily eschews the routine use of antibiotics for growth promotion is thus placed at a competitive disadvantage, which is why may public health experts believe that the problem cannot be solved on an individual basis.

Changes in the way livestock are raised can also lessen the need for antibiotics to treat disease (therapeutic use). Possible changes include raising free-range animals rather than confining them to feeding lots, keeping stock density low and avoiding large herds or flocks, avoiding mixing stocks, following good practices in weaning and transporting animals, and breeding animals for robustness and the ability to resist disease rather than for maximum yield (e.g., faster growth for meat animals or greater production for milk and egg producers). However, these practices also tend to make meat, milk, and egg production more expensive than factory systems, so an individual farmer who chooses to follow them is at a disadvantage compared to those following the current practices of routine antibiotic use.

One argument often made in favor of using antibiotics to promote livestock growth is that the lower production costs results in lower meat, milk, and egg prices for consumers. This argument is often made with reference to industrialized countries such as the United States, although surveys reveal that most Americans already consume at least as much, and frequently more, protein than is recommended for their gender and age group. These dietary practices contrast with the consumption of other types of food, including fruits and vegetables, which are consistently less than recommended in many or all age and gender categories.

Many foods besides meat also contain protein, including legumes, nuts, and seeds, and these foods are typically cheaper than meat. Therefore, even if meat became more expensive, people still would be able to consume a diet with adequate protein. Lower meat consumption also could result in better health because high meat consumption is associated with a number of adverse health outcomes, including increased risk of heart disease, diabetes, and colon cancer, that are not associated with vegetable sources of protein. Increased consumption of meat is also linked to weight gain, and overweight and obesity are associated with many adverse health outcomes, including high blood pressure, high cholesterol, diabetes, stroke, and some types of cancer.

Some individuals, of course, might not be able to afford a healthy diet if the use of antibiotics as livestock growth promoters were banned, just as some people cannot afford a healthy diet today. However, there are many other options to provide assistance to those individuals. One would be to provide financial assistance to people who cannot afford to purchase sufficient, healthy food on their own. Another would be to provide food directly to those individuals. In either case, this assistance would reach the people who are most in need of it, while not requiring the continuation of practices that many experts feel are promoting antibiotic resistance and harming public health.

Developing Countries

The use of antibiotics in food production is a more complex question in developing countries, where food costs are relatively higher and the diets of many individuals may be deficient in protein. On the other hand, the threat to human life of antibiotic-resistant organisms is also greater in developing countries because second- and third-line antibiotics commonly used to treat drug-resistant infections in industrialized countries may not be available in those countries. In addition, these second- and third-line drugs tend to be much more expensive than first-line drugs, so individual patients may not be able to afford them. Finally, because of the greater cost of the second- and third-line drugs, if they are provided by a national health system, they will consume a greater part of the healthcare budget, leaving fewer resources to meet other needs.

Demand for animal sources of protein, including meat and milk, is increasing in many developing and recently industrialized countries. Several factors contribute to this increase, including growing populations, higher incomes that allow the purchase of such foods, and adoption of a more Westernized diet. Methods of meat production are also changing, with the factory farm model commonly used in the United States being adopted by other countries. For instance, an estimated 22 percent of pork in China was produced by factory farm methods in 2007, as compared to 2.5 percent in 1985.

Good measurements of antibiotic use in agriculture or of the prevalence of antibiotic-resistance microorganisms in food-producing animals and meat and dairy products are not available for many countries. However, many experts agree that antibiotic use is increasing and will continue to do so if current policies do not change. For instance, Thomas P. Van Boeckel et al. (2014) estimated that antimicrobial use in livestock production will double in Brazil, China, India, Russia, and South Africa between 2010 and 2030 if current trends continue. China currently consumes 150,000 to 200,000 metric tons of antibiotics annually, about half of which goes into livestock production (mainly pork). Antibiotic pollution of drinking water through agricultural runoff is already a problem in China, with some rivers and city water supplies registering antibiotic levels four times the legal amount required in the United States.

Policy changes in industrialized countries have demonstrated that the reduced use of antibiotics in agriculture need not result in major losses of efficiency or increases in costs, in part due to the savings achieved by not adding antibiotics to feed. Various studies, as cited by O'Neill et al. (1995), have found that the benefits of using antibiotics as growth promoters has declined over the years, to about 5 percent by 2000. In addition, as reported by O'Neill, some countries have enjoyed increased agricultural productivity after reducing or eliminating some uses of antibiotics. For instance, Denmark, one of the largest exporters of pork in the world, increased agricultural productivity by 65 percent from 1992 to 2012, as compared to the European average of 25 percent over the same period, despite having the greatest reduction in agricultural antibiotic use during that time. In the Netherlands, the use of antibiotics as growth promoters was banned in 2006, and 2009 legislation required a 50 percent reduction in total agricultural antibiotic use (including therapeutic use); however, no reduction in productivity or profits was observed between 2009 and 2012. Whether such results will hold in developing countries, where the conditions of production may be different, remains an open question.

SECTION III

Resources

CURRENT REPORTS

ANTIMICROBIAL RESISTANCE: GLOBAL REPORT ON SURVEILLANCE: SUMMARY

Drug resistance is a global problem, and it must be understood at a global level. Unfortunately, there is no international surveillance program in place to gather and process data concerning drug resistance, and many countries also lack a national surveillance program, while data gathered at the local level are not always representative of the population as a whole. The best current source of information regarding drug resistance at the global level is the 2014 report Antimicrobial Resistance: Global Report on Surveillance *from the World Health Organization (WHO). A summary of the report is provided here; the full report presents data from 114 countries on nine bacteria-antibacterial drug combinations of public health significance. While its data have limitations (e.g., only 22 countries provided data on all nine bacteria-antibacterial drug combinations, and some of the data is based on hospital cases only), this report still presents valuable information about drug resistance at the global level.*

Antimicrobial resistance (AMR) is an increasingly serious threat to global public health. AMR develops when a microorganism (bacteria, fungus, virus, or parasite) no longer responds to a drug to which it was originally sensitive. This means that standard treatments no longer work; infections are harder or impossible to control; the risk of the spread of infection to others is increased; illness and hospital stays are prolonged, with added economic and social costs; and the risk of death is greater—in some cases, twice that of patients who have infections caused by non-resistant bacteria.

The problem is so serious that it threatens the achievements of modern medicine. A post-antibiotic era—in which common infections and minor injuries can kill—is a very real possibility for the 21st century.

Determining the scope of the problem is the first step in formulating an effective response to AMR. "Antimicrobial resistance: Global report on surveillance 2014," produced in collaboration with Member States and external partners, is WHO's first attempt to obtain an accurate picture of the magnitude of AMR and the current state of surveillance globally. The report focuses on antibacterial resistance (ABR), as the state of surveillance in ABR is not generally as advanced as it is for diseases such as tuberculosis (TB), malaria, and HIV.

The most important findings of this report are:

- Very high rates of resistance have been observed in all WHO regions in common bacteria (for example, Escherichia coli, Klebsiella pneumoniae and Staphylococcus aureus) that cause common health-care associated and community-acquired infections (urinary tract infections, wound infections, bloodstream infections, and pneumonia).
- Many gaps exist in information on pathogens of major public health importance. There are significant gaps in surveillance, and a lack of standards for methodology, data sharing and coordination. Overall, surveillance of ABR is neither coordinated nor harmonized.

Despite the limitations of current surveillance, it is clear that ABR has reached alarming levels in many parts of the world. There is an urgent need to strengthen and coordinate collaboration to address those gaps. Lessons learned from long-standing experience in TB, malaria and HIV programmes may be usefully applied to ABR and are discussed in the report.

WHO is developing a global action plan for AMR that will include:

- development of tools and standards for harmonized surveillance of ABR in humans, and for integrated surveillance in food-producing animals and the food chain;
- elaboration of strategies for population-based surveillance of AMR and its health and economic impact; and
- collaboration between AMR surveillance networks and centres to create or strengthen coordinated regional and global surveillance.

AMR is a global health security threat that requires action across government sectors and society as a whole. Surveillance that generates reliable data is the essential foundation of global strategies and public health actions to contain AMR.

Key findings and public health implications of ABR are:

- Very high rates of resistance have been observed in bacteria that cause common health-care associated and community-acquired infections (e.g. urinary tract infection, pneumonia) in all WHO regions.

- There are significant gaps in surveillance, and a lack of standards for methodology, data sharing and coordination.

Key findings from AMR surveillance in disease-specific programmes are as follows:

- Although multidrug-resistant TB is a growing concern, it is largely underreported, compromising control efforts.
- Foci of artemisinin resistance in malaria have been identified in a few countries. Further spread, or emergence in other regions, of artemisinin-resistant strains could jeopardize important recent gains in malaria control.
- Increasing levels of transmitted anti-HIV drug resistance have been detected among patients starting antiretroviral treatment.

Surveillance of ABR and sources of data

There is at present no global consensus on methodology and data collection for ABR surveillance. Routine surveillance in most countries is often based on samples taken from patients with severe infections—particularly infections associated with health care, and those in which first-line treatment has failed. Community-acquired infections are almost certainly underrepresented among samples, leading to gaps in coverage of important patient groups.

Nevertheless, it is critical to obtain a broad picture of the international scope of the problem of ABR.

To accomplish this, WHO obtained, from 129 Member States, the most recent information on resistance surveillance and data for a selected set of nine bacteria–antibacterial drug combinations of public health importance. Of these, 114 provided data for at least one of the nine combinations (22 countries provided data on all nine combinations).

Some data sets came from individual surveillance sites, or data from several sources rather than national reports. Many data sets were based on a small number of tested isolates of each bacterium (<30), adding to uncertainty about the precision of the data; this reflects a lack of national structures to provide an overview of the situation and limited capacity for timely information sharing. Most data sets, individual sites or aggregated data, were based on hospital data. Non-representativeness of surveillance data is a limitation for the interpretation and comparison of results.

The data compiled from countries indicate where there may be gaps in knowledge and lack of capacity to collect national data. Among WHO regions, the greatest country-level data were obtained from the European Region and the Region of the Americas, where long-standing regional surveillance and collaboration exist.

Current status of resistance in selected bacteria

In the survey forming the basis for this part of the report, information was requested on resistance to antibacterial drugs commonly used to treat infections caused by seven bacteria of international concern. The chosen bacteria are caus-ing some of the most common infections in different settings; in the community, in hospitals or transmitted through the food chain.

The high proportions of resistance to 3rd-generation cephalosporins reported for E. coli and K. pneumoniae means that treatment of severe infections likely to be caused by these bacteria in many settings must rely on carbapenems, the last-resort to treat severe community and hospital acquired infections. These antibac-terials are more expensive, may not be available in resource-constrained settings, and are also likely to further accelerate development of resistance. Of great con-cern is the fact that K. pneumoniae resistant also to carbapenems has been identi-fied in most of the countries that provided data, with proportions of resistance up to 54% reported. The large gaps in knowledge of the situation in many parts of the world further add to this concern. For E. coli, the high reported resistance to fluo-roquinolones means limitations to available oral treatment for conditions which are common in the community, such as urinary tract infections.

High rates of methicillin-resistant Staphylococcus aureus (MRSA) imply that treatment for suspected or verified severe S. aureus infections, such as common skin and wound infections, must rely on second-line drugs in many countries, and that standard prophylaxis with first-line drugs for orthopaedic and other surgical procedures will have limited effect in many settings. Second-line drugs for S. aureus are more expensive; also, they have severe side-effects for which monitor-ing during treatment is advisable, increasing costs even further.

Reduced susceptibility to penicillin was detected in S. pneumoniae in all WHO regions, and exceeded 50% in some reports. The extent of the problem and its impact on patients is not completely clear because of variation in how the reduced susceptibility or resistance to penicillin is reported, and limited comparability of laboratory standards. Because invasive pneumococcal disease (e.g. pneumonia and meningitis) is a common and serious disease in children and elderly people, better monitoring of this resistance is urgently needed.

The resistance to fluoroquinolones among two of the major causes for bacterial diarrhoea, nontyphoidal Salmonella (NTS) and Shigella species, were compara-tively lower than in E. coli. However, there were considerable gaps in informa-tion on these two bacteria, particularly from areas where they are of major public health importance. Some reports of high resistance in NTS are of great concern because resistant strains have been associated with worse patient outcomes.

In N. gonorrhoeae, finally, decreased susceptibility to third-generation cepha-losporins, the treatment of last resort for gonorrhoea, has been verified in 36 coun-tries and is a growing problem. Surveillance is of poor quality in countries with high disease rates, where there is also a lack of reliable resistance data for gonor-rhoea, and where the extent of spread of resistant gonococci may be high.

Health and economic burden due to ABR

Evidence related to the health and economic burden due to ABR in infections caused by E. coli, K. pneumoniae, and MRSA was examined through systematic reviews of the scientific literature. Patients with infections caused by bacteria resistant to a specific antibacterial drug generally have an increased risk of worse clinical outcomes and death, and consume more health-care resources, than patients infected with the same bacteria not demonstrating the resistance pattern in question. Available data are insufficient to estimate the wider societal impact and economic implications when effective treatment for an infection is completely lost as a result of resistance to all available drugs.

AMR in disease-specific programmes
Tuberculosis
Globally, 3.6% of new TB cases and 20.2% of previously treated cases are estimated to have multidrug-resistant TB (MDR-TB), with much higher rates in Eastern Europe and central Asia. Despite recent progress in the detection and treatment of MDR-TB, the 84 000 cases of MDR-TB notified to WHO in 2012 represented only about 21% of the MDR-TB cases estimated to have emerged in the world that year. Among MDR-TB patients who started treatment in 2010, only 48% (range 46%–56% across WHO regions) were cured after completion of treatment (with 25% lost to follow-up). The treatment success rate was lower among extensively drug-resistant (XDR-TB) cases.

Malaria
Surveillance of antimalarial drug efficacy is critical for the early detection of antimalarial drug resistance, because resistance cannot be detected with routine laboratory procedures. Foci of either suspected or confirmed artemisinin resistance have been identified in Cambodia, Myanmar, Thailand, and Viet Nam. Further spread of artemisinin-resistant strains, or the independent emergence of artemisinin resistance in other regions, could jeopardize important recent gains in malaria control.

HIV
HIV drug resistance is strongly associated with failure to achieve suppression of viral replication and thus with increased risk for disease progression. Data collected between 2004 and 2010 in low- and middle-income countries showed increasing levels of transmitted anti-HIV drug resistance among those starting antiretroviral treatment (ART). Available data suggest that 10%–17% of patients without prior ART in Australia, Europe, Japan, and the United States of America (USA) are infected with virus resistant to at least one antiretroviral drug.

Influenza
Over the past 10 years, antiviral drugs have become important tools for treatment of epidemic and pandemic influenza, and several countries have developed national guidance on their use and have stockpiled the drugs for pandemic preparedness.

However, widespread resistance to adamantanes in currently circulating A(H1N1) and A(H3N2) viruses have left neuraminidase inhibitors as the antiviral agents recommended for influenza prevention and treatment. Although the frequency of oseltamivir resistance in currently circulating A(H1N1)pdm09 viruses is low (1%–2%), the emergence and rapid global spread in 2007/2008 of oseltamivir resistance in the former seasonal A(H1N1) viruses has increased the need for global antiviral resistance surveillance.

AMR in other related areas
Antibacterial resistance in food-producing animals and the food chain

Major gaps exist in surveillance and data sharing related to the emergence of ABR in foodborne bacteria and its potential impact on both animal and human health. Surveillance is hampered by insufficient implementation of harmonized global standards. The multisectoral approach needed to contain ABR includes improved integrated surveillance of ABR in bacteria carried by food-producing animals and in the food chain, and prompt sharing of data. Integrated surveillance systems would enable comparison of data from food-producing animals, food products, and humans.

Resistance in systemic candidiasis

Systemic candidiasis is a common fungal infection worldwide and associated with high rates of morbidity and mortality in certain groups of patients. Although it is known that antifungal resistance imposes a substantial burden on health-care systems in industrialized countries, the global burden of antifungal-resistant Candida is unknown. Resistance to fluconazole, a common antifungal drug, varies widely by country and species. Resistance to the newest class of antifungal agents, the echinocandins, is already emerging in some countries.

Next steps

This report shows major gaps in ABR surveillance, and the urgent need to strengthen collaboration on global AMR surveillance. WHO will therefore facilitate:

- development of tools and standards for harmonized surveillance of ABR in humans, and for integrating that surveillance with surveillance of ABR in food-producing animals and the food chain;
- elaboration of strategies for population-based surveillance of AMR and its health and economic impact; and
- collaboration between AMR surveillance networks and centres to create or strengthen coordinated regional and global surveillance.

AMR is a global health security threat that requires concerted cross-sectional action by governments and society as a whole. Surveillance that generates reliable data is the essential basis of sound global strategies and public health actions to contain AMR, and is urgently needed around the world.

Source: World Health Organization. *Antimicrobial Resistance: Global Report on Surveillance 2014.* Geneva, Switzerland: World Health Organization, 2014. http://www.who.int /drugresistance/documents/surveillancereport/en. Used by permission of the World Health Organization.

ANTIBIOTIC RESISTANCE THREATS IN THE UNITED STATES, 2013: EXECUTIVE SUMMARY

The Centers for Disease Control and Prevention (CDC), located within the U.S. Department of Health and Human Services, provides public health leadership to the United States and works to protect the health, safety, and security of Americans. The 2013 CDC report Antibiotic Resistance Threats in the United States *provides information about antibiotic resistance identified in 18 bacteria, with each classified by level of threat: urgent, serious, or concerning. The executive summary and introduction are provided here; the full report (available from the CDC web site: www.cdc.gov) also describes efforts to prevent and counter the threat posed by antibiotic resistance, including four core actions: preventing infections and resistant bacteria from spreading, tracking resistant bacteria, improving use of antibiotics, and promoting the development of new antibiotics and diagnostic tests. A third section of the report includes information about what different stakeholders, including communities, healthcare workers, patients, states, and the CDC, can do to combat antibiotic resistance. A reference section includes a glossary, technical information, and references for sources of further information.*

Antibiotic Resistance Threats in the United States, 2013 is a snapshot of the complex problem of antibiotic resistance today and the potentially catastrophic consequences of inaction.

The overriding purpose of this report is to increase awareness of the threat that antibiotic resistance poses and to encourage immediate action to address the threat. This document can serve as a reference for anyone looking for information about antibiotic resistance. It is specifically designed to be accessible to many audiences. For more technical information, references and links are provided.

This report covers bacteria causing severe human infections and the antibiotics used to treat those infections. In addition, Candida, a fungus that commonly causes serious illness, especially among hospital patients, is included because it, too, is showing increasing resistance to the drugs used for treatment. When discussing the pathogens included in this report, Candida will be included when referencing "bacteria" for simplicity. Also, infections caused by the bacteria Clostridium difficile (C. difficile) are also included in this report. Although C. difficile infections are not yet significantly resistant to the drugs used to treat them, most are directly related to antibiotic use and thousands of Americans are affected each year.

Drug resistance related to viruses such as HIV and influenza is not included, nor is drug resistance among parasites such as those that cause malaria. These are important problems but are beyond the scope of this report. The report consists of multiple one or two page summaries of cross-cutting and bacteria-specific antibiotic resistance topics. The first section provides context and an overview of antibiotic resistance in the United States. In addition to giving a national assessment of the most dangerous antibiotic resistance threats, it summarizes what is known about the burden of illness, level of concern, and antibiotics left to defend against these infections. This first section also includes some basic background information, such as fact sheets about antibiotic safety and the harmful impact that resistance can have on high-risk groups, including those with chronic illnesses such as cancer.

CDC estimates that in the United States, more than two million people are sickened every year with antibiotic-resistant infections, with at least 23,000 dying as a result. The estimates are based on conservative assumptions and are likely minimum estimates. They are the best approximations that can be derived from currently available data.

Regarding level of concern, CDC has—for the first time—prioritized bacteria in this report into one of three categories: urgent, serious, and concerning.

Urgent Threats
- Clostridium difficile
- Carbapenem-resistant Enterobacteriaceae (CRE)
- Drug-resistant Neisseria gonorrhoeae

Serious Threats
- Multidrug-resistant Acinetobacter
- Drug-resistant Campylobacter
- Fluconazole-resistant Candida (a fungus)
- Extended spectrum β-lactamase producing Enterobacteriaceae (ESBLs)
- Vancomycin-resistant Enterococcus (VRE)
- Multidrug-resistant Pseudomonas aeruginosa
- Drug-resistant Non-typhoidal Salmonella
- Drug-resistant Salmonella Typhi
- Drug-resistant Shigella
- Methicillin-resistant Staphylococcus aureus (MRSA)
- Drug-resistant Streptococcus pneumoniae
- Drug-resistant tuberculosis

Concerning Threats
- Vancomycin-resistant Staphylococcus aureus (VRSA)
- Erythromycin-resistant Group A Streptococcus
- Clindamycin-resistant Group B Streptococcus

The second section describes what can be done to combat this growing threat, including information on current CDC initiatives. Four core actions that fight the spread of antibiotic resistance are presented and explained, including 1) preventing infections from occurring and preventing resistant bacteria from spreading, 2) tracking resistant bacteria, 3) improving the use of antibiotics, and 4) promoting the development of new antibiotics and new diagnostic tests for resistant bacteria.

The third section provides summaries of each of the bacteria in this report. These summaries can aid in discussions about each bacteria, how to manage infections, and implications for public health. They also highlight the similarities and differences among the many different types of infections.

This section also includes information about what groups such as states, communities, doctors, nurses, patients, and CDC can do to combat antibiotic resistance. Preventing the spread of antibiotic resistance can only be achieved with widespread engagement, especially among leaders in clinical medicine, healthcare leadership, agriculture, and public health. Although some people are at greater risk than others, no one can completely avoid the risk of antibiotic-resistant infections. Only through concerted commitment and action will the nation ever be able to succeed in reducing this threat.

A reference section provides technical information, a glossary, and additional resources.

Any comments and suggestions that would improve the usefulness of future publications are appreciated and should be sent to Director, Division of Healthcare Quality Promotion, National Center for Emerging and Zoonotic Infectious Diseases, Centers for Disease Control and Prevention, 1600 Clifton Road, Mailstop A-07, Atlanta, Georgia, 30333. E-mail can also be used: hip@cdc.gov.

Source: Centers for Disease Control and Prevention. "Antibiotic Resistance Threats in the United States, 2013." http://www.cdc.gov/drugresistance/pdf/ar-threats-2013-508.pdf (accessed April 26, 2015).

ANTIMICROBIAL RESISTANCE SURVEILLANCE IN EUROPE, 2015: SUMMARY

Comparing rates of antibiotic resistance in different countries can be very instructive, particularly if the countries are similar economically, culturally, and geographically and the quality of data is similar across countries. This type of comparison is facilitated by Antibiotic Resistance in the European Union, *a report prepared annually by the European Centre for Disease Prevention and Control. The 2015 report is based on data reported in 2014 by 29 European countries, including all members of the European Union except for Poland, and two countries in the European Economic Area (Iceland and Norway). The summary, which is included here, presents information about four organisms:* Klebsiella pneumoniae, Escherichia coli Acetinobactor *species, and Meticillin-resistant* Staphylococcus aureus *(MRSA;* meticillin *is another name for methicillin), with maps and statistics to facilitate comparisons in the rates and spread of antibiotic-resistance between countries and between the years 2011 and 2014. The full report, available from the web site of the European Centre for Disease Prevention and Control, (http://ecdc.europa.eu/en/Pages/home.aspx), includes more detailed information.*

Summary of the latest data on antibiotic resistance in the European Union EARS-Net surveillance data, November 2015

- Antibiotic resistance is a serious threat to public health in Europe, leading to increased healthcare costs, prolonged hospital stays, treatment failures, and sometimes death.
- Over the last four years (2011–2014), the percentages of *K. pneumoniae* resistant to fluoroquinolones, third-generation cephalosporins and aminoglycosides, as well as combined resistance to all three antibiotic groups, has increased significantly at EU/EEA level.
- During the same period, resistance to third-generation cephalosporins and combined resistance to fluoroquinolones, third-generation cephalosporins, and aminoglycosides in *E. coli* increased significantly at EU/EEA level.
- Carbapenems are an important group of last-line antibiotics for treatment of infections involving multidrug-resistant gram-negative bacteria such as *K. pneumoniae* and *E. coli.* Although carbapenem resistance remains at relatively low levels for most countries, the significant increase of the population-weighted EU/EEA mean percentage of carbapenem resistance in *K. pneumoniae* is a cause for serious concern and a threat to patient safety in Europe.
- Antibiotic resistance in Acinetobacter species shows large intercountry variations in Europe. High percentages of isolates with combined resistance to fluoroquinolones, aminoglycosides, and carbapenems were reported from the Baltic countries, southern and southeastern Europe.
- In countries with high levels of multidrug resistance, including resistance to carbapenems, only a few therapeutic options are available, for example polymyxins. In these countries, the large number of isolates with resistance to polymyxins is an important warning that options for the treatment of infected patients are becoming even more limited.
- The percentage of meticillin-resistant *Staphylococcus aureus* showed a significantly decreasing trend at EU/EEA level between 2011 and 2014, but the decrease was less pronounced compared to the period 2009 to 2012.
- Prudent antibiotic use and comprehensive infection prevention and control strategies targeting all healthcare sectors (acute care hospitals, long-term care facilities, and ambulatory care) are the cornerstones of effective interventions to prevent selection and transmission of antibiotic-resistant bacteria.

Antibiotic resistance in the European Union

The data presented in this section were collected by the European Antimicrobial Resistance Surveillance Network (EARS-Net), which is coordinated by ECDC. For 2014, a total of 29 countries, including all EU Member States except Poland, and two EEA countries (Iceland and Norway), reported data to EARS-Net. For more details on EARS-Net, surveillance results, and information on methods, please refer to the EARS-Net Annual Report 2014 and the EARS-Net interactive database.

Klebsiella pneumoniae

Klebsiella pneumoniae is a common cause of urinary tract, respiratory tract, and bloodstream infections. It can spread rapidly between patients in healthcare settings and is a frequent cause of hospital outbreaks.

Antibiotic resistance in *K. pneumoniae* is a public health concern of increasing importance in Europe. More than one third of the *K. pneumoniae* isolates reported to EARS-Net for 2014 were resistant to at least one antibiotic group under surveillance, and resistance to multiple antibiotic groups was common.

The EU/EEA population-weighted mean percentages of *K. pneumoniae* resistant to fluoroquinolones, third-generation cephalosporins, aminoglycosides, and combined resistance to all three of these antibiotic groups increased significantly between 2011 and 2014. The increasing trend of combined resistance to fluoroquinolones, third-generation cephalosporins, and aminoglycosides from 16.7% in 2011 to 19.6% in 2014 means that for patients who are infected with these multidrug-resistant bacteria, only few therapeutic options remain available. Among these are the carbapenems, a last-line group of antibiotics.

Although carbapenem-resistance percentages remained at low levels for most countries in 2014, resistance to carbapenems at EU/EEA level significantly increased over the last four years, from a population-weighted mean percentage of 6.0% in 2011 to 7.3% in 2014. Resistance to carbapenems was more frequently reported in *K. pneumoniae* bloodstream infections from south and southeastern Europe than from other parts of Europe.

Very few therapeutic options are left for patients infected with multidrug-resistant *K. pneumoniae* with additional resistance to carbapenems, and are often limited to combination therapy and to older antibiotics such as polymyxins. Although data on polymyxin susceptibility as part of EARS-Net surveillance are not complete, the fact that some countries, especially countries with already high percentages of carbapenem resistance, report large numbers of isolates with polymyxin resistance is an indication of the further loss of effective treatment options for gram-negative bacterial infections.

Escherichia coli

Escherichia coli is one of the most frequent causes of bloodstream infections and community- and healthcare-associated urinary tract infections worldwide.

Antibiotic resistance in *E. coli* requires close attention as the percentages of isolates resistant to commonly used antibiotics continue to increase throughout

Europe. More than half of the isolates reported to EARS-Net in 2014 were resistant to at least one antibiotic group under surveillance.

Of particular concern is the increase in resistance to third-generation cephalosporin, which increased significantly on EU/EEA level from 9.6% in 2011 to 12.0% in 2014, and combined resistance to third-generation cephalosporins, fluoroquinolones, and aminoglycosides, which increased significantly on EU/EEA level from 3.8% in 2011 to 4.8% in 2014. Several countries reported statistically significant increasing trends for these types of resistance during the period 2011 to 2014.

Resistance to carbapenems in *E. coli* remains low in Europe.

Acinetobacter species

Acinetobacter species mainly cause healthcare-associated infections, such as pneumonia and bloodstream infections, and often results in hospital outbreaks.

Antibiotic resistance in *Acinetobacter* spp. showed large variations across Europe, with generally very high resistance percentages reported from the Baltic countries, southern and southeastern Europe. Combined resistance to fluoroquinolones, aminoglycosides, and carbapenems was the most frequently reported resistance phenotype in 2014 and accounted for almost half of the reported isolates. Eight out of 25 countries reporting susceptibility results for 10 or more isolates had percentages for this type of combined resistance of 50% or higher, indicating seriously limited options for the treatment of patients infected with *Acinetobacter* spp. in these countries.

Resistance to polymyxins was observed in 4% of the isolates, with a vast majority reported from southern Europe. These results should be interpreted with caution due to the low number of isolates tested and differences in laboratory methodology to determine susceptibility. However, the high levels of resistance to multiple antibiotics reported from several places in Europe is of great concern, especially when resistance to carbapenems is already high and resistance to polymyxins starts being reported.

Meticillin-resistant *Staphylococcus aureus*

Meticillin-resistant *Staphylococcus aureus* (MRSA) is one of the most frequent causes of antibiotic-resistant, healthcare-associated infections worldwide. In addition, increasing levels of community-associated MRSA are being reported from many parts of the world, including Europe.

As in previous years, large intercountry variations in MRSA percentages were observed across Europe in 2014, with percentages ranging from 0.9 % to 56%. The EU/EEA population-weighted mean percentage decreased significantly from 18.6% in 2011 to 17.4% in 2014, but the decrease was less pronounced, compared with that observed for the period 2009 to 2012.

Comprehensive MRSA strategies targeting all healthcare sectors (acute, long-term care facilities, and ambulatory care) remain essential to sustain the reduction of the spread of MRSA in Europe.

Source: European Centre for Disease Prevention and Control. "Summary of the latest data on antibiotic resistances in the European Union: 2015." (Nov. 18, 2015). http://ecdc.europa .eu/en/eaad/antibiotics-get-informed/antibiotics-resistance-consumption/Documents /antibiotics-resistance-EU-data-2015.pdf (accessed July 11, 2016).

POLICY STATEMENTS

WHO GLOBAL STRATEGY FOR CONTAINMENT OF ANTIMICROBIAL RESISTANCE: EXECUTIVE SUMMARY

In 1998, the World Health Assembly of the WHO passed a resolution urging member-states to develop ways to combat antimicrobial resistance. Similar concerns prompted the WHO in 2011 to issue the WHO Global Strategy for Containment of Antimicrobial Resistance: Executive Summary, *which synthesizes the available information to provide a framework of interventions to guide individual countries in their efforts to slow the emergence of antimicrobial-resistant microorganisms and to reduce their spread. The executive summary of this document is included here; the full document is available from the WHO web site (www.who .int). Separate sections recommend specific actions that can be performed by different groups of people and organizations, including patients and the general community, prescribers and dispensers, hospitals, pharmaceutical manufacturers, people involved in caring for food-producing animals, national governments and health systems, people involved in drug and vaccine development, and people involved with pharmaceutical promotion. A final section considers actions that can be taken at the international level to combat antimicrobial resistance.*

- Deaths from acute respiratory infections, diarrhoeal diseases, measles, AIDS, malaria and tuberculosis account for more than 85% of the mortality from infection worldwide. Resistance to first-line drugs in most of the pathogens causing these diseases ranges from zero to almost 100%. In some instances, resistance to second- and third-line agents is seriously compromising treatment outcome. Added to this is the significant global burden of resistant hospital-acquired infections, the emerging problems of antiviral resistance and the increasing problems of drug resistance in the neglected parasitic diseases of poor and marginalized populations.
- Resistance is not a new phenomenon; it was recognized early as a scientific curiosity and then as a threat to effective treatment outcome. However, the development of new families of antimicrobials throughout the 1950s and 1960s and of modifications of these molecules through the 1970s and 1980s allowed us to believe that we could always remain ahead of the pathogens. By the turn of the century, this complacency had come to haunt us. The pipeline of new drugs is running dry and the incentives to develop new antimicrobials to address the global problems of drug resistance are weak.

- Resistance costs money, livelihoods and lives and threatens to undermine the effectiveness of health delivery programmes. It has recently been described as a threat to global stability and national security. A few studies have suggested that resistant clones can be replaced by susceptible ones; in general, however, resistance is slow to reverse or is irreversible.
- Antimicrobial use is the key driver of resistance. Paradoxically this selective pressure comes from a combination of overuse in many parts of the world, particularly for minor infections, misuse due to lack of access to appropriate treatment and underuse due to lack of financial support to complete treatment courses.
- Resistance is only just beginning to be considered as a societal issue and, in economic terms, as a negative externality in the health care context. Individual decisions to use antimicrobials (taken by the consumer alone or by the decision-making combination of health care worker and patient) often ignore the societal perspective and the perspective of the health service.
- The World Health Assembly (WHA) Resolution of 1998[1] urged Member States to develop measures to encourage appropriate and cost-effective use of antimicrobials, to prohibit the dispensing of antimicrobials without the prescription of a qualified health care professional, to improve practices to prevent the spread of infection and thereby the spread of resistant pathogens, to strengthen legislation to prevent the manufacture, sale and distribution of counterfeit anti-microbials and the sale of antimicrobials on the informal market, and to reduce the use of antimicrobials in food-animal production. Countries were also encouraged to develop sustainable systems to detect resistant pathogens, to monitor volumes and patterns of use of antimicrobials and the impact of control measures.
- Since the WHA Resolution, many countries have expressed growing concern about the problem of antimicrobial resistance and some have developed national action plans to address the problem. Despite the mass of literature on anti-microbial resistance, there is depressingly little on the true costs of resistance and the effectiveness of interventions. Given this lack of data in the face of a growing realization that actions need to be taken now to avert future disaster, the challenge is *what to do* and *how to do it*.
- The WHO Global Strategy for Containment of Antimicrobial Resistance addresses this challenge. It provides a framework of interventions to slow the emergence and reduce the spread of antimicrobial-resistant microorganisms through:
  - reducing the disease burden and the spread of infection
  - improving access to appropriate antimicrobials
  - improving use of antimicrobials

1. World Health Organization. World Health Assembly (fifty-first). *Emerging and other communicable diseases: antimicrobial resistance.* WHA51.17, 1998, agenda item 21.3.

- strengthening health systems and their surveillance capabilities
- enforcing regulations and legislation
- encouraging the development of appropriate new drugs and vaccines.
- The strategy highlights aspects of the containment of resistance and the need for further research directed towards filling the existing gaps in knowledge.
- The strategy is people-centred, with interventions directed towards the groups of people who are involved in the problem and need to be part of the solution, i.e. prescribers and dispensers, veterinarians, consumers, policy-makers in hospitals, public health and agriculture, professional societies and the pharmaceutical industry.
- The strategy addresses antimicrobial resistance in general rather than through a disease-specific approach, but is particularly focused on resistance to antibacterial drugs.
- Much of the responsibility for implementation of the strategy will fall on individual countries. Governments have a critical role to play in the provision of public goods such as information, in surveillance, analysis of cost-effectiveness and cross-sectoral coordination.
- Given the complex nature of antimicrobial resistance, the strategy necessarily contains a large number of recommendations for interventions. Prioritization of the implementation of these interventions needs to be customized to national realities. To assist in this process, an implementation approach has been defined together with indicators for monitoring implementation and outcomes.
- Recognition that the problem of resistance exists and the creation of effective national intersectoral task forces are considered critical to the success of implementation and monitoring of interventions. International interdisciplinary cooperation will also be essential.
- Improving antimicrobial use must be a key action in efforts to contain resistance. This requires improving access and changing behaviour; such changes take time.
- Containment will require significant strengthening of the health systems in many countries and the costs of implementation will not be negligible. However, such costs must be weighed against future costs averted by the containment of widespread antimicrobial resistance.

Summary of recommendations for intervention

Patients and the general community and prescribers and dispensers

The emergence of antimicrobial resistance is a complex problem driven by many interconnected factors, in particular the use and misuse of antimicrobials. Antimicrobial use, in turn, is influenced by an interplay of the knowledge, expectations, and interactions of prescribers and patients, economic incentives, characteristics of the health system(s), and the regulatory environment. In the light of this complexity, coordinated interventions are needed that simultaneously target the behaviour of providers and patients and change important features of the environments in which they interact. These interventions are most likely to be successful if the following factors are understood within each health setting:

—which infectious diseases and resistance problems are important
—which antimicrobials are used and by whom
—what factors determine patterns of antimicrobial use
—what the relative costs and benefits are from changing use
—what barriers exist to changing use.

Although the interventions directed towards providers and patients are presented separately (1 and 2) for clarity, they will require implementation in an integrated fashion.

1. PATIENTS AND THE GENERAL COMMUNITY
Education
  1.1 Educate patients and the general community on the appropriate use of antimicrobials.
  1.2 Educate patients on the importance of measures to prevent infection, such as immunization, vector control, use of bednets, etc.
  1.3 Educate patients on simple measures that may reduce transmission of infection in the household and community, such as handwashing, food hygiene, etc.
  1.4 Encourage appropriate and informed health care seeking behaviour.
  1.5 Educate patients on suitable alternatives to anti-microbials for relief of symptoms and discourage patient self-initiation of treatment, except in specific circumstances.

2. PRESCRIBERS AND DISPENSERS
Education
  2.1 Educate all groups of prescribers and dispensers (including drug sellers) on the importance of appropriate antimicrobial use and containment of antimicrobial resistance.
  2.2 Educate all groups of prescribers on disease prevention (including immunization) and infection control issues.
  2.3 Promote targeted undergraduate and postgraduate educational programmes on the accurate diagnosis and management of common infections for all health care workers, veterinarians, prescribers, and dispensers.
  2.4 Encourage prescribers and dispensers to educate patients on antimicrobial use and the importance of adherence to prescribed treatments.

2.5 Educate all groups of prescribers and dispensers on factors that may strongly influence their prescribing habits, such as economic incentives, promotional activities, and inducements by the pharmaceutical industry.

Management, guidelines, and formularies

2.6 Improve antimicrobial use by supervision and support of clinical practices, especially diagnostic and treatment strategies.

2.7 Audit prescribing and dispensing practices and utilize peer group or external standard comparisons to provide feedback and endorsement of appropriate anti-microbial prescribing.

2.8 Encourage development and use of guidelines and treatment algorithms to foster appropriate use of antimicrobials.

2.9 Empower formulary managers to limit antimicrobial use to the prescription of an appropriate range of selected antimicrobials.

Regulation

2.10 Link professional registration requirements for prescribers and dispensers to requirements for training and continuing education.

Hospitals

Although most antimicrobial use occurs in the community, the intensity of use in hospitals is far higher; hospitals are therefore particularly important in the containment of anti-microbial resistance. In hospitals, it is crucial to develop integrated approaches to improving the use of antimicrobials, reducing the incidence and spread of hospital-acquired (nosocomial) infections, and linking therapeutic and drug supply decision-making. This will require training of key individuals and the allocation of resources to effective surveillance, infection control, and therapeutic support.

3. HOSPITALS

Management

3.1 Establish infection control programmes, based on current best practice, with the responsibility for effective management of antimicrobial resistance in hospitals and ensure that all hospitals have access to such a programme.

3.2 Establish effective hospital therapeutics committees with the responsibility for overseeing antimicrobial use in hospitals.

3.3 Develop and regularly update guidelines for antimicrobial treatment and prophylaxis, and hospital antimicrobial formularies.

3.4 Monitor antimicrobial usage, including the quantity and patterns of use, and feedback results to prescribers.

Diagnostic laboratories

3.5 Ensure access to microbiology laboratory services that match the level of the hospital, e.g. secondary, tertiary.

3.6 Ensure performance and quality assurance of appropriate diagnostic tests, microbial identification, anti-microbial susceptibility tests of key pathogens, and timely and relevant reporting of results.

3.7 Ensure that laboratory data are recorded, preferably on a database, and are used to produce clinically- and epidemiologically-useful surveillance reports of resistance patterns among common pathogens and infections in a timely manner with feedback to prescribers and to the infection control programme.

Interactions with the pharmaceutical industry

3.8 Control and monitor pharmaceutical company promotional activities within the hospital environment and ensure that such activities have educational benefit.

Use of antimicrobials in food-producing animals

A growing body of evidence establishes a link between the use of antimicrobials in food-producing animals and the emergence of resistance among common pathogens. Such resistance has an impact on animal health and on human health if these pathogens enter the food chain. The factors affecting such antimicrobial use, whether for therapeutic, prophylactic or growth promotion purposes, are complex and the required interventions need coordinated implementation. The underlying principles of appropriate antimicrobial use and containment of resistance are similar to those applicable to humans. The WHO global principles for the containment of antimicrobial resistance in animals intended for food[2] were adopted at a WHO consultation in June 2000 in Geneva. They provide a framework of recommendations to reduce the overuse and misuse of antimicrobials in food animals for the protection of human health. Antimicrobials are widely used in a variety of other settings outside human medicine, e.g. horticulture and aquaculture, but the risks to human health from such uses are less well understood and they have not been included in this document.

4. USE OF ANTIMICROBIALS IN FOOD-PRODUCING ANIMALS

This topic has been the subject of specific consultations, which resulted in "WHO global principles for the containment of antimicrobial resistance in animals intended for food."[3] A complete description of all recommendations is contained in that document, and only a summary is reproduced here.

---

2. World Health Organization. *WHO global principles for the containment of antimicrobial resistance in animals intended for food.* 2000. www.who.int emc/diseases/zoo/who_global_principles.html

3. World Health Organization. *WHO global principles for the containment of antimicrobial resistance in animals intended for food.* 2000. www.who.int emc/diseases/zoo/who_global_principles.html

Summary

4.1 Require obligatory prescriptions for all antimicrobials used for disease control in food animals.

4.2 In the absence of a public health safety evaluation, terminate or rapidly phase out the use of antimicrobials for growth promotion if they are also used for treatment of humans.

4.3 Create national systems to monitor antimicrobial usage in food animals.

4.4 Introduce pre-licensing safety evaluation of anti-microbials with consideration of potential resistance to human drugs.

4.5 Monitor resistance to identify emerging health problems and take timely corrective actions to protect human health.

4.6 Develop guidelines for veterinarians to reduce overuse and misuse of antimicrobials in food animals.

National governments and health systems

Government health policies and the health care systems in which they are implemented play a crucial role in determining the efficacy of interventions to contain antimicrobial resistance. National commitment to understand and address the problem and the designation of authority and responsibility are prerequisites. Effective action requires the introduction and enforcement of appropriate regulations and allocation of appropriate resources for education and surveillance. Constructive interactions with the pharmaceutical industry are critical, both for ensuring appropriate licensure, promotion, and marketing of existing antimicrobials and for encouraging the development of new drugs and vaccines. For clarity, interventions relating to these interactions with the industry are shown in separate recommendation groups (6 and 7).

5.1 Introduce legal requirements for manufacturers to collect and report data on antimicrobial distribution (including import/export).

5.2 Create economic incentives for the appropriate use of antimicrobials.

Policies and guidelines

5.3 Establish and maintain updated national Standard Treatment Guidelines (STGs) and encourage their implementation.

5.4 Establish an Essential Drugs List (EDL) consistent with the national STGs and ensure the accessibility and quality of these drugs.

5.5 Enhance immunization coverage and other disease preventive measures, thereby reducing the need for antimicrobials.

Education

5.6 Maximize and maintain the effectiveness of the EDL and STGs by conducting appropriate undergraduate and postgraduate education programmes of health care professionals on the importance of appropriate anti-microbial use and containment of antimicrobial resistance.

5.7 Ensure that prescribers have access to approved prescribing literature on individual drugs.

Surveillance of resistance, antimicrobial usage, and disease burden

5.8 Designate or develop reference microbiology laboratory facilities to coordinate effective epidemiologically sound surveillance of antimicrobial resistance among common pathogens in the community, hospitals, and other health care facilities. The standard of these laboratory facilities should be at least at the level of recommendation 3.6.

5.9 Introduce legal requirements for manufacturers to collect and report data on antimicrobial distribution (including import/export).

5.10 Create economic incentives for the appropriate use of antimicrobials.

6. PHARMACEUTICAL PROMOTION

6.1 Introduce requirements for pharmaceutical companies to comply with national or international codes of practice on promotional activities.

6.2 Ensure that national or international codes of practice cover direct-to-consumer advertising, including advertising on the Internet.

6.3 Institute systems for monitoring compliance with legislation on promotional activities.

6.4 Identify and eliminate economic incentives that encourage inappropriate antimicrobial use.

6.5 Make prescribers aware that promotion in accordance with the datasheet may not necessarily constitute appropriate antimicrobial use.

7. INTERNATIONAL ASPECTS OF CONTAINING ANTIMICROBIAL RESISTANCE

7.1 Encourage collaboration between governments, non-governmental organizations, professional societies, and international agencies to recognize the importance of antimicrobial resistance, to present consistent, simple, and accurate messages regarding the importance of antimicrobial use, antimicrobial resistance, and its containment, and to implement strategies to contain resistance.

7.2 Consider the information derived from the surveillance of antimicrobial use and antimicrobial resistance, including the containment thereof, as global public goods for health to which all governments should contribute.

7.3 Encourage governments, non-governmental organizations, professional societies and international agencies to support the establishment of networks, with trained staff and adequate infrastructures, which can undertake epidemiologically valid surveillance of antimicrobial resistance and antimicrobial use to provide information for the optimal containment of resistance.

Source: World Health Organization. *WHO Global Strategy for Containment of Antimicrobial Resistance: Executive Summary*. Geneva, Switzerland: World Health Organization, 2001. http://www.who.int/drugresistance/WHO_Global_Strategy_English.pdf (accessed July 11, 2016). Used by permission of the World Health Organization.

NATIONAL STRATEGY FOR COMBATING ANTIBIOTIC RESISTANT BACTERIA: EXECUTIVE SUMMARY

In September 2014, the White House issued the policy document "National Strategy for Combating Antibiotic-Resistant Bacteria," which was part of an national effort to combat the growth and spread of antibiotic-resistant bacteria in the United States; other aspects of this national effort include a 2014 Executive Order on Combating Antibiotic Resistance issued by President Barack Obama, and a National Action Plan approved in 2014 that directs federal agencies to accelerate their response to this growing threat. The executive summary and introduction of the "National Strategy" document are included here; the complete document is available from the White House web site (www.whitehouse.gov). This document reviews the threat that antibiotic resistance poses to the nation's health and outlines five goals for action to combat it: slow the emergence and prevent of spread of resistant organisms; strengthen national surveillance networks; develop and use rapid and innovative diagnostic tests to identify and characterize resistant bacteria; accelerate basic and applied research and development for new antibiotics, therapeutics, and vaccines; and improve international cooperation and collaboration.

Executive Summary

The discovery of antibiotics in the early 20th century fundamentally transformed human and veterinary medicine. Antibiotics now save millions of lives each year in the United States and around the world. The rise of antibiotic-resistant bacterial strains, however, represents a serious threat to public health and the economy. The Centers for Disease Control and Prevention (CDC) estimates that annually, at least two million illnesses and 23,000 deaths are caused by antibiotic-resistant bacteria in the United States alone.[4] If the effectiveness of antibiotics (drugs that kill or inhibit the growth of bacteria) is lost, we will no longer be able to reliably and rapidly treat bacterial infections, including bacterial pneumonias, foodborne illnesses, and healthcare-associated infections. As more strains of bacteria become resistant to an ever-larger number of antibiotics, our drug choices have become increasingly limited and more expensive and, in some cases, nonexistent. In a world with few effective antibiotics, modern medical advances such as surgery, transplants, and chemotherapy may no longer be viable due to the threat of infection.

The *National Strategy for Combating Antibiotic Resistant Bacteria* identifies priorities and coordinates investments: to prevent, detect, and control outbreaks of resistant pathogens recognized by CDC as urgent or serious threats, including carbapenem-resistant *Enterobacteriaceae* (CRE), methicillin-resistant *Staphylococcus aureus* (MRSA), ceftriaxone-resistant *Neisseria gonorrhoeae*, and *Clostridium difficile,* which is naturally resistant to many drugs used to treat other

---

4. Centers for Disease Control and Prevention. *Antibiotic Resistance Threats in the United States, 2013* (http://www.cdc.gov/drugresistance/threat-report-2013/)

infections and proliferates following administration of antibiotics; to ensure continued availability of effective therapies for the treatment of bacterial infections; and to detect and control newly resistant bacteria that emerge in humans or animals. This *National Strategy* is the basis of a 2014 Executive Order on Combating Antibiotic Resistance, as well as a forthcoming *National Action Plan* that directs Federal agencies to accelerate our response to this growing threat to the nation's health and security. The *National Action Plan* will be informed by a report approved by the President's Council of Advisors on Science and Technology (PCAST) on July 11, 2014.

The *National Strategy* outlines five interrelated goals for action by the United States Government in collaboration with partners in healthcare, public health, veterinary medicine, agriculture, food safety, and academic, Federal, and industrial research. The goals include:

Slow the Emergence of Resistant Bacteria and Prevent the Spread of Resistant Infections. Judicious use of antibiotics in healthcare and agricultural settings is essential to slow the emergence of resistance and extend the useful lifetime of effective antibiotics. Antibiotics are a precious resource, and preserving their usefulness will require cooperation and engagement by healthcare providers, healthcare leaders, pharmaceutical companies, veterinarians, the agricultural industry, and patients. Effective dissemination of information to the public is critical. Prevention of resistance also requires rapid detection and control of outbreaks, along with regional efforts to control transmission across community and healthcare settings.

1. **Strengthen National One-Health Surveillance Efforts to Combat Resistance.** Antibiotic resistance can arise in bacterial pathogens affecting humans, animals, and the environment. Strengthening detection and control of resistance requires the adoption of a "One-Health" approach that promotes integration of public health and veterinary disease, food, and environmental surveillance. Improved detection can be achieved through appropriate data sharing, enhancement, expansion, and coordination of existing surveillance systems, and creation of a regional laboratory network that provides a standardized platform for resistance testing and advanced capacity for genetic characterization of bacteria, including whole genome sequencing.

2. **Advance Development and Use of Rapid and Innovative Diagnostic Tests for Identification and Characterization of Resistant Bacteria.** Today, researchers are taking advantage of new technologies to develop rapid "point-of-need" tests that can be used during a healthcare visit to distinguish between viral and bacterial infections and identify bacterial drug susceptibilities—an innovation that could significantly reduce unnecessary antibiotic use. The availability of new rapid diagnostic tests, combined with ongoing use of culture-based assays to identify new resistance mechanisms, will advance the detection and control of resistant bacteria.

3. **Accelerate Basic and Applied Research and Development for New Antibiotics, Other Therapeutics, and Vaccines.** Antibiotics that lose their effectiveness for treating human disease through antibiotic resistance must be replaced with new drugs. Alternatives to antibiotics are also needed in agriculture and veterinary medicine. The advancement of drug development requires intensified efforts to boost basic scientific research, facilitate clinical trials of new antibiotics, attract greater private investment, and increase the number of antibiotic drug candidates in the drug-development pipeline. We must also promote the development of other tools to combat resistance, including new and next-generation antibiotics, vaccines, additional therapeutics, and diagnostics.

4. **Improve International Collaboration and Capacities for Antibiotic Resistance Prevention, Surveillance, Control, and Antibiotic Research and Development.** Recognized by G8 Science Ministers in 2013 as "a major health security challenge of the 21st century," antibiotic resistance is a global problem that requires global solutions. The United States will work in concert with the World Health Organization (WHO), the Food and Agriculture Organization of the United Nations (FAO), the World Organization for Animal Health (OIE), ministries of health and agriculture, and other domestic and international stakeholders to strengthen national and international capacities to detect, monitor, analyze, report and characterize antibiotic resistance; provide resources and incentives to spur the development of therapeutics and diagnostics for use in humans and animals; and strengthen regional networks and global partnerships that help prevent and control the emergence and spread of resistance. The United States will support the development of the WHO *Global Action Plan* to address antimicrobial resistance, strengthen cooperation under the European Union-United States Trans-Atlantic Task Force on Antimicrobial Resistance, promote antibiotic resistance as an international health priority, and mobilize resources for global activities through multilateral venues such as the Global Health Security Agenda.

Introduction

The discovery of antibiotics in the early 20th century fundamentally transformed human and veterinary medicine. Antibiotics now save millions of lives each year in the United States and around the world. The rise of antibiotic-resistant bacterial strains, however, represents a serious threat to public health and the economy. The CDC estimates that annually at least two million illnesses and 23,000 deaths are caused by antibiotic-resistant bacteria in the United States alone.

As more strains of bacteria become resistant to an ever-larger number of antibiotics, our drug choices will become increasingly limited and expensive and, in some cases, nonexistent. If this trend continues unchecked, a wide range of modern medical procedures, from basic dental care to organ transplants, likely would be accompanied by a much greater risk of developing a difficult-to-treat or untreatable antibiotic infection. The safety of many modern medical procedures is dependent on the ability to treat bacterial infections that can arise as post-treatment complications.

Scope of the *National Strategy:* "Antibiotic resistance" results from mutations or acquisition of new genes in bacteria that reduce or eliminate the effectiveness of antibiotics. "Antimicrobial resistance" is a broader term that encompasses resistance to drugs to treat infections caused by many different types of pathogens, including bacteria, viruses (e.g., influenza and the human immunodeficiency virus (HIV), parasites (e.g., the parasitic protozoan that causes malaria), and fungi (e.g., *Candida spp.*). While all of these pathogens are dangerous to human health, this *Strategy* focuses on resistance in bacteria that presents a serious or urgent threat to public health.

Guiding Principles

Our approach to combating the emergence and spread of antibiotic resistant bacteria takes into consideration goals and objectives including the following:

- Misuse and over-use of antibiotics in healthcare and food production continue to hasten the development of bacterial drug resistance, leading to loss of efficacy of existing antibiotics;
- Detecting and controlling antibiotic resistance requires the adoption of a "One-Health" approach to disease surveillance that recognizes that resistance can arise in humans, animals, and the environment;
- Implementation of evidence-based infection control practices can prevent the spread of resistant pathogens;
- Interventions are necessary to accelerate private sector investment in the development of therapeutics to treat bacterial infections because current private sector interest in antibiotic development is limited;
- There are opportunities to use innovations and new technologies—including whole-genome sequencing, metagenomics, and bioinformatic approaches—to develop next-generation tools to strengthen human and animal health, including:
  - Point-of-need diagnostic tests to distinguish rapidly between bacterial and viral infections as well as identify bacterial drug susceptibilities;
  - New antibiotics and other therapies that provide much needed treatment options for those infected with resistant bacterial strains;
- Antibiotic resistance is a global health problem that requires international attention and collaboration, because bacteria do not recognize borders.

Goals and Objectives

With these principles in mind, the *Strategy* lays out five interrelated goals that guide collaborative action by the U.S. Government in partnership with foreign governments, individuals, and organizations aiming to strengthen healthcare, public health, veterinary medicine, agriculture, food safety, and research and manufacturing. Those goals include:

1. Slow the emergence of resistant bacteria and prevent the spread of resistant infections;
2. Strengthen national One-Health surveillance efforts to combat resistance;
3. Advance development and use of rapid and innovative diagnostic tests for identification and characterization of resistant bacteria;
4. Accelerate basic and applied research and development for new antibiotics, other therapeutics, and vaccines; and
5. Improve international collaboration and capacities for antibiotic-resistance prevention, surveillance, control, and antibiotic research and development.

. . . Development and implementation of the *National Strategy* also supports World Health Assembly (WHA) resolution 67.25 (Antimicrobial Resistance), which was endorsed in May 2014, and urges countries to develop and finance national plans and strategies and take urgent action at the national, regional, and local levels to combat resistance. The resolution specifically calls on WHA Member States to develop practical and feasible approaches to extend the lifespan of drugs, strengthen pharmaceutical management systems and laboratory infrastructure, develop effective surveillance systems, and encourage the development of new diagnostics, drugs, and treatment options.

Development of the Strategy

In December 2013, the President directed the National Security Council (NSC) and the Office of Science and Technology Policy (OSTP) to assess the current and growing threat of antibiotic resistance and develop a multi-sectoral plan to combat resistant bacteria. NSC and OSTP established an interagency policy committee to review past and current Federal efforts to address antibiotic resistance. The committee—which included representatives from the Department of Health and Human Services (HHS), the Department of Agriculture (USDA), the Departments of Homeland Security (DHS), State, Defense (DOD), Veterans Affairs (VA), the U.S. Agency for International Development (USAID), and the Environmental Protection Agency (EPA)—suggested practical, evidence-based ways to enhance antibiotic stewardship, strengthen surveillance for antibiotic resistance and use, advance the development of new diagnostics, antibiotics, and novel therapies, and accelerate research and innovation. The results of the review provided the basis for this *National Strategy*.

Partnerships and Implementation

The *National Strategy for Combating Antibiotic-Resistant Bacteria* will be implemented in accordance with a forthcoming *National Action Plan*, which will detail specific steps and milestones for achieving the *Strategy*'s goals and objectives along with metrics for measuring progress. The *National Action Plan* will also address recommendations made in the PCAST *Report to the President on Combating Antibiotic Resistance.*

Implementation of the *National Action Plan* will require the sustained, coordinated, and complementary efforts of individuals and groups around the world, including many who will contribute to its development. These include public and private sector partners, healthcare providers, healthcare leaders, veterinarians, agriculture industry leaders, manufacturers, policymakers, and patients. All of us who depend on antibiotics must join in a common effort to detect, stop, and prevent the emergence and spread of resistant bacteria.

Source: The White House. "National Strategy for Combating Antibiotic-Resistant Bacteria." (September 2014). https://www.whitehouse.gov/sites/default/files/docs/carb_national _strategy.pdf (accessed July 11, 2016).

THE JUDICIOUS USE OF MEDICALLY IMPORTANT ANTIMICROBIAL DRUGS IN FOOD-PRODUCING ANIMALS: EXECUTIVE SUMMARY

In 2012, the Center for Veterinary Medicine of the FDA issued "The Judicious Use of Medically Important Antimicrobial Drugs in Food-Producing Animals," a nonbinding document in its Guidance for Industry *series. This document provides an overview of the problem of antimicrobial resistance, with a particular focus on the use of medically important antimicrobial drugs in food-producing animals, summarizes the current FDA regulatory framework, summarizes the FDA's current activities with regard to this issue, and issues recommendations for combating antimicrobial resistance. Two principles guide these recommendations: (1) medically important antimicrobial drugs should be used in food-producing animals only as necessary to protect the animals' health, and (2) such drugs should be used in food-producing animals only under veterinary oversight or consultation. The executive summary and excerpts from this report are included here; the full document, which also includes a historical summary of the FDA's actions with regard to the use of antibiotics in agriculture and summaries of key reports and relevant peer-reviewed research, is available from the FDA web site (www.fda.gov).*

I. Executive Summary

Antimicrobial drugs have been widely used in human and veterinary medicine for more than 50 years, with tremendous benefits to both human and animal health. The development of resistance to this important class of drugs, and the resulting loss of their effectiveness as antimicrobial therapies, poses a serious public health threat. Misuse and overuse of antimicrobial drugs creates selective evolutionary pressure that enables antimicrobial resistant bacteria to increase in numbers more rapidly than antimicrobial susceptible bacteria and thus increases the opportunity for individuals to become infected by resistant bacteria.

Because antimicrobial drug use contributes to the emergence of drug resistant organisms, these important drugs must be used judiciously in both animal and human medicine to slow the development of resistance. Efforts have been made to promote the judicious use of these drugs in humans (see http://www.cdc.gov /getsmart/index.html) as well as in animals (see http://www.avma.org/issues/default .asp). Using these drugs judiciously means that unnecessary or inappropriate use should be avoided. The focus of this document is on the use of medically important antimicrobial drugs[5] in food-producing animals. Based on a consideration of the available scientific information, FDA is providing a framework for the voluntary adoption of practices to ensure the appropriate or judicious use of medically important antimicrobial drugs in food-producing animals. This framework includes the principles of phasing in such measures as 1) limiting medically important antimicrobial drugs to uses in food-producing animals that are considered necessary for assuring animal health; and 2) limiting such drugs to uses in food-producing animals that include veterinary oversight or consultation. Developing strategies for reducing antimicrobial resistance is critically important for protecting both public and animal health. Collaboration involving the public, the public health, animal health, and animal agriculture communities on the development and implementation of such strategies is needed to assure that the public health is protected while also assuring that such strategies are feasible and that the health needs of animals are addressed.

FDA's guidance documents, including this guidance, do not establish legally enforceable responsibilities. Instead, guidances describe the Agency's current thinking on a topic and should be viewed only as recommendations, unless specific regulatory or statutory requirements are cited. The use of the word "should" in Agency guidances means that something is suggested or recommended, but not required.

I. Introduction

Antimicrobial resistance[6], and the resulting failure of antimicrobial therapies in humans, is a mounting public health problem of global significance. This phenomenon is driven by many factors, including the use of antimicrobial drugs in

---

5. The term "medically important antimicrobial drugs" generally refers to antimicrobial drugs that are important for therapeutic use in humans.

6. The term "antimicrobial" refers broadly to drugs with activity against a variety of microorganisms including bacteria, viruses, fungi, and parasites. Antimicrobial drugs that have specific activity against bacteria are referred to as antibacterial or antibiotic drugs. However, the broader term "antimicrobial," commonly used in reference to drugs with activity against bacteria, is used in this document interchangeably with the terms antibacterial or antibiotic. Antimicrobial resistance is the ability of bacteria or other microbes to resist the effects of a drug. Antimicrobial resistance, as it relates to bacterial organisms, occurs when

both humans and animals. In regard to animal use, this document addresses the use of medically important antimicrobial drugs in food-producing animals for production or growth-enhancing purposes. These uses, referred to as production[7] uses throughout this document, are typically administered through the feed or water on a herd- or flock-wide basis and are approved for such uses as increasing rate of weight gain or improving feed efficiency.

Unlike other uses of these drugs in animals (e.g., for the treatment, control, and prevention of disease), these "production uses" are not intended to manage a specific disease that may be ongoing or at risk of occurring, but rather are expressly indicated and used for the purpose of enhancing the production of animal-derived products (e.g., increasing rate of weight gain or improving feed efficiency). This document summarizes some of the key reports and scientific literature related to the use of antimicrobial drugs in animal agriculture and outlines FDA's current thinking on strategies for assuring that medically important antimicrobial drugs are used judiciously in food-producing animals in order to help minimize antimicrobial resistance development. In finalizing this guidance, FDA has considered comments that were submitted to the docket, and other relevant information. If you have additional relevant information, please submit it to the docket at any time. We are particularly interested in any new information regarding the use of medically important antimicrobials in food-producing animals and its impact on the development of drug-resistant bacteria.

II. Current Regulatory Framework

FDA considers the issue of antimicrobial resistance as part of its human food safety review related to new animal drugs used in food-producing animals. FDA considers an antimicrobial new animal drug to be "safe" if the agency concludes that there is "reasonable certainty of no harm to human health" from the proposed use of the drug in food-producing animals. This standard applies to safety evaluations completed prior to new animal drug approvals, as well as to those completed for drugs after approval. If this safety standard is not met before approval, the drug cannot be approved. If safety issues arise after approval, the Federal Food, Drug, and Cosmetic Act (the Act) provides grounds for withdrawal of approval of new animal drug applications for safety reasons. For example, section 512(e)(1)(B) of the Act provides for withdrawal of new animal drug application approvals when new evidence, along with evidence contained in the application, shows that the drug is not shown to be safe under the approved conditions of use. Under this provision, if FDA initiates a withdrawal action, it must produce evidence to show that there is a reasonable basis from which serious questions may be inferred about

---

bacteria change in some way that reduces or eliminates the effectiveness of drugs, chemicals, or other agents designed to treat bacterial infections.

7. Production uses are also referred to as "nontherapeutic" or "subtherapeutic" uses, terms that we believe lack sufficient clarity.

the ultimate safety of the drug and any substance that may be formed in or on food as a result of use of such drug under approved conditions. Once the agency meets this initial burden, the burden then shifts to the sponsor to demonstrate the safety of the drug (Docket no. 00N-1571, at p. 5, Mar. 16, 2004).

In 2003, FDA implemented new policies for evaluating antimicrobial resistance associated with use of antimicrobial new animal drugs in food-producing animals through the issuance of Guidance for Industry (GFI) #152, "Evaluating the Safety of Antimicrobial New Animal Drugs with Regard to their Microbiological Effects on Bacteria of Human Health Concern" (http://www.fda.gov/downloads /AnimalVeterinary/GuidanceComplianceEnforcement/GuidanceforIndustry /UCM052519.pdf). This guidance document describes a risk-based assessment process for evaluating antimicrobial resistance associated with the use of antimicrobial new animal drugs in food-producing animals. The guidance also recommends measures for mitigating such risk.

In general, FDA's GFI #152 is premised on the concept that increasing the exposure of bacterial populations to antimicrobial drugs increases the risk of generating resistance to those antimicrobial drugs. Pursuant to this principle, the administration of medically important antimicrobial drugs to entire herds or flocks of food-producing animals (e.g., for production purposes) would represent a use that poses a qualitatively higher risk to public health than the administration of such drugs to individual animals or targeted groups of animals (e.g., to prevent, control, or treat specific diseases). In addition to factors that impact the potential extent of use of the drug, the guidance also considers such factors as the properties of the drug in question including mechanism of action and mechanism of resistance, the prevalence of zoonotic foodborne bacteria in the food-producing animal species for which the drug is intended, and the importance of the drug in question as a therapy in humans. Risk-mitigating factors that are considered include such limitations as restricting use of the drug to use by or on the order of a veterinarian.

Although FDA developed GFI #152 primarily to assess antimicrobial resistance risks as part of the new animal drug approval process, the underlying concept described above is also applicable to safety evaluations conducted for previously-approved antimicrobial new animal drugs. Therefore, FDA considers this same concept when it conducts safety evaluations for currently approved antimicrobial drugs, including those approved for use in animal feed.

From a practical standpoint, however, some significant differences exist between applying the GFI #152 risk assessment approach to the pre-approval process and applying it to safety reviews of currently-approved products. On the pre-approval side, the GFI #152 assessment process, including the various risk mitigation measures described, is taken into consideration by drug sponsors upstream in the drug development process and, in effect, steers product development in a direction that is most consistent with the guidance. On the post-approval side, FDA may examine certain currently-approved products to determine whether such products appear consistent with GFI #152. However, initiating action to withdraw an approved new animal drug application (NADA), in whole or in part, based on the results of a post-approval safety review would require the agency to make the showing required under section 512(e)(1) of the Act.

Alternatively, concerns associated with approved NADAs can sometimes be addressed through more informal processes. For example, in certain cases FDA has worked collaboratively with the sponsor of an NADA to address concerns raised regarding their product and has initiated steps to permit the sponsor to voluntarily withdraw part or all of the NADA or to revise the product labeling to address the concern. This alternative pathway can in some cases be an effective and expedient mechanism for resolving issues associated with an NADA.

III. Status of FDA's Current Activities

In general, the antimicrobial new animal drug applications that FDA is addressing as part of its efforts to evaluate the public health concerns associated with the use of medically important antimicrobial drugs in food-producing animals can be divided into two broad categories: 1) those NADAs submitted after the issuance of GFI #152 in 2003 and for which FDA is assessing the microbiological safety of the new animal drug on a pre-approval basis using the principles outlined in GFI #152; and 2) those NADAs approved before the final version of GFI#152 was issued in 2003. In regard to the first category, FDA believes the approach outlined in GFI #152 for evaluating microbiological safety as part of the drug approval process has been very effective. As noted above, that assessment process and the associated risk mitigation measures are usually taken into consideration by industry during the drug development process. Thus, products that ultimately move forward toward approval are those products that include use conditions that are consistent with the guidance and are intended to minimize the extent to which product use would contribute to resistance development.

FDA believes the approach outlined in GFI #152 is scientifically sound and is protective of the public health. FDA recognizes that the list of drugs in Appendix A is not static and should be periodically reassessed and updated as necessary. Such reassessment is necessary to take into consideration such factors as the development of new antimicrobials for human therapy, the emergence of diseases in humans, or changes in prescribing practices in the United States. FDA will update Appendix A, as necessary, through a separate process that will also be subject to public comment.

The second category of products [is] those antimicrobial NADAs that were approved prior to the implementation of GFI #152. Some of the products in this category include products that were approved for use in food-producing animals more than 30 years ago. Of particular concern, as discussed in section IV, are those products that are approved for use in animal feed for production or growth-enhancing purposes. Although these products are FDA-approved, their approval occurred prior to implementation of current processes for assessing safety with respect to antimicrobial resistance. Furthermore, the scientific understanding regarding antimicrobial resistance has advanced significantly over this time frame and, as discussed earlier in this document, a number of scientific reports have raised public health concerns regarding the use of medically important antimicrobials in food-producing animals.

As a result, FDA is examining available information regarding medically important antimicrobial drugs currently approved for use in food-producing animals and considering potential steps for agency action.

IV. Recommended Principles Regarding Judicious Use in Animals

The continued availability of effective antimicrobial drugs is critically important for combating infectious disease in both humans and animals. This includes the continued availability of feed and water uses of such drugs for managing disease in animal agriculture. Therefore, it is in the interest of both human and animal health that we take a more proactive approach to considering how antimicrobial drugs are being used, and take steps to assure that such uses are appropriate and necessary for maintaining the health of humans and animals. Using medically important antimicrobial drugs as judiciously as possible is key to minimizing resistance development and preserving the effectiveness of these drugs as therapies for humans and animals. Although FDA applauds the efforts to date by various veterinary and animal producer organizations to institute guidelines for the judicious use of antimicrobial drugs, the agency believes additional, voluntary steps are needed.

To further address this public and animal health concern, FDA is recommending two additional principles about the appropriate or judicious use of medically important antimicrobial drugs in food-producing animals. These principles are consistent with the recommendations of a number of recent scientific panels or committees referenced earlier in this document including the 1997, 2000, and 2011 reports of the WHO, the 2003 IOM Report, and the 2005 Codex Code of Practice.

FDA recognizes the need to collaborate with the animal health and animal producer communities on strategies for minimizing animal health impacts or industry disruption that may be associated with the implementation of changes by animal drug sponsors to voluntarily align the use conditions of affected drug products with the principles outlined below. Furthermore, FDA intends to consult with the United States Department of Agriculture (USDA) on implementation strategies, including the development of a framework for veterinary oversight and consultation requirements. FDA is committed to assuring that the public health is protected while also assuring that the health needs of animals are addressed.

Principle 1: *The use of medically important antimicrobial drugs in food-producing animals should be limited to those uses that are considered necessary for assuring animal health.*

In light of the risk that antimicrobial resistance poses to public health, FDA believes the use of medically important antimicrobial drugs in food-producing animals for production purposes (e.g., to promote growth or improve feed efficiency) represents an injudicious use of these important drugs. Production uses are not directed at any specifically identified disease, but rather are expressly indicated and used for the purpose of enhancing the production of animal-derived products. In contrast, FDA considers uses that are associated with the treatment, control, or prevention[8] of specific diseases, including administration through feed or water, to be uses that are necessary for assuring the health of food-producing animals.

Some may have concerns that the use of medically important antimicrobial drugs in food-producing animals for disease prevention purposes is not an appropriate or judicious use. However, FDA believes that some indications for prevention use are necessary and judicious as long as such use includes professional veterinary involvement. Veterinary involvement in the decision-making process associated with the use of medically important antimicrobial drugs is an important aspect of assuring appropriate use, including judicious prevention use. When determining the appropriateness of a prevention use, veterinarians consider several important factors such as determining the medical rationale for such use, and that such use is appropriately targeted at a specific etiologic agent and appropriately timed relative to the disease. For example, if a veterinarian determines, based on the client's production practices and herd health history, that cattle being transported or otherwise stressed are more likely to develop a certain bacterial infection, preventively treating these cattle with an antimicrobial approved for prevention of that bacterial infection would be considered a judicious use. Another example would be the prevention of necrotic enteritis in broiler chickens. In this case, the prevention use of an antimicrobial is important to manage this disease in certain flocks in the face of concurrent coccidiosis, a significant parasitic disease in chickens. On the other hand, FDA would not consider the administration of a drug to apparently healthy animals in the absence of any information that such animals were at risk of a specific disease to be a judicious use. The decision to use a specific drug or combination drug is generally based on factors that veterinarians are uniquely qualified to consider, including the mode of antibacterial action, drug distribution in specific tissues, and the duration of effective drug levels at the site of infection.

Principle 2: *The use of medically important antimicrobial drugs in food-producing animals should be limited to those uses that include veterinary oversight or consultation.*

Most of the feed-use antimicrobial drugs are currently approved for over-the-counter use in food-producing animals for purposes that include the treatment,

---

8. Disease prevention involves the administration of an antimicrobial drug to animals, none of which are exhibiting clinical signs of disease, in a situation where disease is likely to occur if the drug is not administered.

control, and prevention of disease as well as for production purposes (i.e., for growth promotion uses such as increased rate of weight gain). In addition to instituting voluntary measures that would limit use of medically important antimicrobial drugs in food-producing animals to uses that are considered necessary to assure the animals' health, FDA also believes it is important to phase-in the voluntary practice of including veterinary oversight or consultation in the use of these drugs. As noted above, FDA believes that this practice is an important mechanism for helping to assure appropriate use. Veterinarians can play a critical role in the diagnosis of disease and in the decision-making process related to instituting measures to treat, control, or prevent disease. FDA recognizes that the nature of veterinary involvement can vary due to numerous factors such as geographic location and animal production setting. In fact, there are limited numbers of large animal veterinarians, which can make consultation or oversight challenging in certain situations. For example, some animal disease events require immediate attention. In some cases, veterinarians may be directly diagnosing and administering therapies, while in other cases they are visiting and consulting with producers periodically to establish customized disease management protocols for that producer's herd or flock. Of key importance to FDA is the fact that, in both of these cases, the veterinarian is involved in the decision-making process regarding antimicrobial drug use. FDA recognizes that increasing veterinary involvement in the use of antimicrobial drugs has significant practical implications for animal producers, veterinary practitioners, and the veterinary profession as whole. Therefore, FDA is particularly interested in receiving comments on strategies for effectively promoting the voluntary adoption of such a change.

V. Conclusion

In order to minimize the development of antimicrobial resistance, FDA believes that it is important to ensure the judicious use of medically important antimicrobial drugs in animal agriculture. We recommend several steps to accomplish this including voluntary measures that would limit medically important antimicrobial drugs to uses in food-producing animals that are considered necessary for assuring animal health and that include veterinary oversight or consultation. Such limitations would reduce overall medically important antimicrobial drug use levels, thereby reducing antimicrobial resistance selection pressure, while still maintaining the availability of these drugs for appropriate use.

Source: Center for Veterinary Medicine, U.S. Food and Drug Administration. "The Judicious Use of Medically Important Antimicrobial Drugs in Food-Producing Animals." Guidance for Industry #209. (April 13, 2012). http://www.fda.gov/downloads/AnimalVeteri nary/GuidanceComplianceEnforcement/GuidanceforIndustry/UCM216936.pdf (accessed July 11, 2016).

TIMELINE

1632–1723   Lifetime of Antonie van Leeuwenhoek, who was the first to observe single-celled microorganisms (e.g., protozoa and bacteria), which he called *animalicula*.

1818–1865   Lifetime of Ignaz Semmelweis, a Hungarian physician who promoted the practice of hand washing in obstetric clinics, a practice which substantially reduced the incidence of puerperal fever (also known as *childbed fever*) among women giving birth.

1822–1895   Lifetime of Louis Pasteur, who demonstrated that microorganisms could contaminate liquids, and concluded that they could infect humans as well.

1827–1912   Lifetime of Joseph Lister, an English surgeon who promoted the use of antiseptic procedures in surgery, including the use of carbolic acid to sterilize surgical instruments.

1853–1938   Lifetime of Christian Gram, a Danish chemist who developed the Gram stain technique for identifying bacteria.

1881–1955   Lifetime of Sir Alexander Fleming, a Scottish biologist credited with the isolation of penicillin, and recipient of the 1945 Nobel Prize in Physiology or Medicine (shared with Howard Walter Florey and Ernest Boris Chain).

1896   British bacteriologist Ernest Hankin reports that the waters of the Ganges and Jumna rivers in India display antibacterial activity against *Vibrio cholerae*, the bacterium that causes cholera.

1905   The German scientist Robert Heinrich Herman Koch (1843–1910) is awarded the Nobel Prize in Physiology or Medicine for his work on tuberculosis. Koch also studied cholera and developed Koch's postulates, a series of principles to determine if a microorganism caused a particular disease. Although no longer applied strictly as Koch stated them, these postulates were an important step in developing the germ theory of disease.

1909   The first modern chemotherapeutic agent is introduced into medicine. Salversan, also called Compound 606, was synthesized by Paul Ehrlich and his research team in Germany and is used to treat syphilis. The development of Salversan was a product of Ehrlich's ideal of discovering medicine that would work like a "magic bullet" by attacking a disease without harming other parts of the body.

1910   The existence of bacteriophages, viruses that kill bacteria, is discovered by French microbiologist Felix d'Herelle in Mexico. Although some credit the English bacteriologist Frederick Twort with the discovery of bacteriophages several years earlier, Twort did not follow up on his observations, and thus d'Herelle is often credited with the discovery of bacteriophages.

1919   d'Herelle successfully uses bacteriophages to treat dysentery at the *Hôpital des Enfants-Malades* in Paris; before administering the phages to patients, d'Herelle and several staff members consumed them to test their safety.

1932   The first sulfa drug, Prontosil, is introduced into medical care (it was discovered in 1932). Prontosil is effective against Gram-positive bacteria by inhibiting dihydropteroate synthase, an enzyme in the bacteria.

1938   Penicillin, the first drug in the beta-lactam (β-lactam) class, is introduced into medical care (it was discovered in 1928). Penicillin is a broad-spectrum antibiotic that works by inhibiting cell wall biosynthesis.

1938   The federal Food, Drug, and Cosmetic Act is passed in the United States, giving the Food and Drug Administration (FDA) authority to regulate drug safety. Passage of this law was motivated largely by an incident in which over 100 children in the United States were killed by Elixire Sulfanilamide, a toxic remedy containing sulfanilamide in diethylene glycol.

1939   Gerhard J. P. Domagk is awarded the Nobel Prize in Physiology or Medicine for his work in developing Prontosil and other sulfa drugs while working at I.G. Farben. The Nazi government then ruling Germany did not allow Domagk to receive the Nobel Prize at that time, but he was able to receive it in 1947 following Germany's defeat in World War II.

1940s   In animal husbandry, the ability of subclinical doses of antibiotics in feed to promote animal growth is discovered.

1942   Resistance to Prontosil, the first sulfa drug, is first observed.

1944   Chlortetracycline, a broad-spectrum antibiotic and the first of the tetracycline class of antibiotics, is discovered and introduced into medical care.

1945   Resistance to penicillin, a broad-spectrum antibiotic of the β-lactam class, is observed.

1945   The Nobel Prize in Physiology or Medicine is awarded jointly to Fleming, Florey, and Chain for their work on penicillin.

1946   Streptomycin, the first antibiotic in the aminoglycoside class, is introduced into medical care (it had been discovered in 1943). It is a broad-spectrum antibiotic and the first antibiotic to be effective against tuberculosis (TB). The same year, bacterial resistance to streptomycin is observed.

1948   Chloramphenicol, a broad-spectrum antibiotic, is introduced into medical care (it had been discovered in 1946).

1949   Penicillin is incorporated as an element in the plot of Carol Reed's film *The Third Man*. In it, Orson Welles plays a character who sells penicillin on the black market in postwar Vienna, but in concentrations too weak to be effective in treating disease.

1950   Resistance to chloramphenicol, a broad-spectrum antibiotic, is observed.

1950s   The United States approved the use of antibiotics in animal husbandry as growth promoters.

1951   Erythromycin, the first of the macrolide class of antibiotics, is introduced into medical care (it was discovered in 1957). Erythromycin is effective against Gram-positive bacteria.

1952   Resistance to chlortetracycline, a broad-spectrum antibiotic, is observed.

1952   Selman A. Waksman is awarded the Nobel Prize in Physiology or Medicine for his work in discovering antibiotics through the screening of soil bacteria and fungi. Antibiotics discovered in this way include streptomycin, the first antibiotic effective against TB; actinomycin; and neomycin.

1958   Rifampicin, the first of the rifamycin class of antibiotics, in introduced into medical care (it had been discovered the previous year). Rifampicin is effective against Gram-positive bacteria.

1958   Vancomycin, the first drug in the glycopeptide class of anti-biotics, is introduced into medical care (it had been discovered in 1953). Vancomysin is effective against Gram-positive bacteria and works by inhibiting cell wall biothesynthesis.

1960   Resistance to vancomysin is observed.

1962   Resistance to erythromycin and rifampicin is observed.

1964   Dorothy C. Hodgkin is awarded the Nobel Prize in Chemistry for her work in X-ray crystallography. One of her accomplishments was discovering penicillin, around 1944.

1968   Ciprofloxacin, the first of the quinolone class of antibiotics, is introduced into medical care (it had been discovered in 1961). Ciprofloxacin is a broad-spectrum antibiotic that works by inhibiting DNA synthesis. Resistance to ciprofloxacin is observed the same year.

1969   In the United Kingdom, the Swann Committee links the use of antibiotics as growth promoters in animal husbandry to the emergence of resistant strains of bacteria. The committee also divides antimicrobials into two classes—those used as therapeutic agents and that require a prescription, and those used as feed additives without a prescription—and recommended restricting the use of antibiotics as animal growth promoters.

1976   Stuart Levy and colleagues at the Tufts University School of Medicine (in Medford, Massachusetts) demonstrate that antibiotic resistance can be spread from animals to humans. Specifically, they demonstrate that multidrug-resistant strains of *E. coli* found in chickens were also detected in people living near the chickens, although the humans were not taking any antibiotics.

1980s Ruth Hummel, Wolfgang Witte, and Helmut Tschápe, working at the Robert Koch Institute in East Germany, demonstrate that bacteria resistant to the antibiotic streptomycin could be transferred from animals to humans.

1986   Sweden becomes the first country to ban the use of antibiotics as growth promoters in animal food production.

1988   The Institute of Medicine, part of the National Academies of the United States, issues a report identifying the growth of antibiotic resistance through the use of antibiotics as animal growth promoters as a hazard.

1997   A meeting of the World Health Organization (WHO) in Berlin, organized around the topic "The medical impact of the use of antibiotics in food animals," results in a call for the cessation of the use of medically important antimicrobials as animal growth promoters.

1997   The European Union bans the use of avoparcin for agricultural uses, following evidence that vancomycin-resistant *Enterococcus* (VRE), detected in human patients, was also present in the meat and waste products of animals on farms where avoparcin was used as a growth promoter.

1998   Streptogramin B, the first of the streptogramin class of antibiotics, is introduced into medical care (it had been discovered in 1963). The long delay between introduction and discovery was because the streptogramins (i.e., Streptogramin A and B), which are generally used together, present some difficulties in use, but they became clinically important in the late 1990s because they are effective against some bacteria that have developed resistance to other antibiotics.

1999   Several organizations, including the Center for Science in the Public Interest, the Food Animal Concern Trust, Public Citizen, and the Union of Concerned Scientists, file a petition requesting the FDA to ban the use of antibiotics as animal growth promoters.

1999   The European Union bans several classes of antibiotics important in human medicine from use as growth promoters in animal husbandry; drugs banned at this time include tylosin, spiramycin, virginiamycin, and bacitracin.

2000   Linezolid, an antbiotic of the oxazolidinone class, is introduced into medical care. The primary use of linezolid, which was discovered in 1955, is to treat infections with Gram-posiitive bacteria resistant to other antibiotics.

2001   The European Surveillance of Antimicrobial Consumption is created to gather data about the use of antimicrobials in medical care.

2003   Daptomycin, an antibiotic of the lipopeptide class, is introduced into medical care. Discovered in 1966, it is used to treat infections with Gram-positive bacteria that are resistant to several other antibiotics.

2003   The Institute of Medicine issues a second report stating that evidence suggests a relationship between bacterial resistance in humans and use of antibiotics in animal husbandry.

2003   The FDA issues nonbinding guidelines stating that medically important antibiotics are unlikely to be approved for use as food additives for animal husbandry, but the guidelines do not affect the antibiotics already approved for that purpose.

2005   The FDA bans the use of fluoroquinolones, a class of antibiotics important in human medicine, for use in poultry production.

2005   Several organizations, including the American Public Health Organization, the American Academy of Pediatrics, and the Union of Concerned Scientists, ask the FDA to ban the use of all medically important antibiotics, including those already approved as growth promoters, from agricultural use.

2006   The European Union bans the use of all antimicrobials as growth promoters in agriculture.

2008   The European Surveillance of Veterinary Antimicrobial Consumption Project requests that the European Medicines Agency harmonize surveillance programs for collecting data on the sales and usage of antimicrobials.

2011   Fidaxomycin, a narrow-spectrum antibiotic of the macrolide class, in introduced into medical care. Fidaxomycin is effective against Gram-positive bacteria and is used to treat infections with *Clostridium difficile*; it works by inhibiting RNA polymerase.

2012   Bedaquiline, an antibiotic of the diarylquinoline class, is introduced into medical care. Discovered in 1997, it is a narrow-spectrum antibiotic used to treat infections with multidrug-resistant tuberculosis (MDR-TB).

June 2013   The Phagoburn project begins in Europe, with funding by the European Commission, for the purpose of investigating the use of phage therapy (therapy with viruses that kill bacteria) for burns infected with *E. coli* and *Pseudomonas aeruginosa*.

June 2014   Research led by Barry Marshall of the University of Western Australia finds that *Helicobacter pylori*, a bacteria that causes ulcers in humans, can mutate quickly in the first weeks of infection to evade the body's immune system.

June 2014   A research team led by Kjersti Aagaard of Texas Children's Hospital and the Baylor College of Medicine found that bacteria can reach unborn children through the placenta. The bacteria identified in the study were not disease-causing, but of the types that normally reside in human bodies.

July 2014   A study in China finds that the recycled water (treated sewage) used to irrigate city parks in seven cities found that this practice may expose many people to antibiotic-resistant germs. The parks watered using recycled water were found to contain as much as 8,655 times the microbial antibiotic resistance genes as those parks watered with fresh water.

September 2014   Researchers led by Martin Blaser of New York University discover that the use of antibiotics in infant mice resulted in obesity in adult animals. The mechanism believed responsible for this result is alterations in the animals' gut microbiome, the community of microbes living in their intestines.

October 2014   A study by researchers from the Vanderbilt University Medical Center in Nashville, Tennessee, found that American college athletes playing contact sports such as American football were more than twice as likely to have methicillin resistant *S. aureus* (MRSA) bacteria in their bodies than college students participating in noncontact sports such as track and field.

October 2014   Antibiotic-resistant superbugs are included among a list of "real-life Halloween horrors in the natural world" published by *Science News*.

December 2014   A paper by a research team led by Joshua Wallace at the University of Buffalo, delivered at the annual meeting of the Society of Environmental Toxicology, reported that 2013 flooding in Colorado spread antibiotic-resistant microbes to water supplies, including river headwaters, that previously had been free of them.

December 2014   A study found that people with high levels of the antimicrobial triclosan, included in many products such as hand soap and toothpaste, are more likely to also harbor *S. aureus* bacteria in their noses. Because of the potential for *S. aureus* to cause serious infections, including pneumonia, the FDA began reviewing the use of triclosan in personal care products such as soap.

January 2015   Scientists at Texas Tech University find that antibiotic-resistant bacteria can be transmitted from cattle to humans over distances through the wind. The study looked at the levels of veterinary antibiotics in downwind and upwind samples of 10 high-density cattle facilities near Lubbock, Texas; that area was studied because of its dry and windy climate, which produced ideal conditions for the transmission of antibiotics by the wind.

March 2015   The White House issues the *National Action Plan for Combating Antibiotic Resistant Bacteria*. Among other things, this report calls for reducing the use in antibiotics in animal husbandry and inappropriate antibiotics prescribing in medicine, and requiring hospitals and medical clinics to develop programs to fight antimicrobial resistance.

March 2015   Scientists from the University of Exeter (United Kingdom) report the existence of *E. coli* bacteria resistance to third-generation cephalosporins (an antibiotic class used to treat many types of infections in humans) on the surface of Britain's coastal waters. Although the proportion of resistant bacteria was low (0.12 percent on average) and the resistant bacteria were found at only a minority of sites sampled (15 of 97 sites), this discovery is a cause for concern, as swimmers could contract drug-resistant infections from these waters.

April 2015 A study found that workers on pig farms in Iowa were six times as likely as those not having regular contact with pigs to carry drug-resistant bacteria, including MRSA.

May 2015 A typhoid epidemic in Africa is traced to a drug-resistant H58 strain of the typhoid bacterium *Salmonella typhi*, which was first noted in South Asia 25 to 30 years earlier and also has been identified in the Middle East and Pacific Islands. The H58 strain was found most often in Africa, in areas where older antibiotics are frequently used to treat typhoid.

June 2015 The Australian health minister, Sussan Ley, announces a national campaign to end the overuse of antibiotics in both humans and livestock.

August 2015 The National Institute of Health and Care Excellence (United Kingdom) issues a report stating that doctors in England write about 10 million unnecessary antibiotic prescriptions annually, and that about one in four cases when such a prescription is written, antibiotics are not medically necessary for the patient.

October 2015 California passes legislation, which will go into effect in January 2018, banning the use of antibiotics as growth promoters in animal husbandry; this legislation is the strictest yet passed in the United States.

December 2015 Dame Sally Davies, the chief medical officer of England, warns that due to drug resistance, gonorrhea is in danger of becoming an untreatable disease. Her warning was in part prompted by an outbreak of "super-gonorrhea," a strain resistant to azithromycin, with 16 cases of infection by it reported between March and December 2015.

March 2016 A study by researchers at the Imperial College London and Bristol University found that in about 50 percent of pediatric cases of urinary tract infections (UTIs) in the 26 countries studied, the bacteria causing the infection had become resistant to commonly prescribed antibiotics.

May 2016 The CDC reports a case in Pennsylvania of a patient infected by a strain of *E. coli* resistant to colistin, currently used as a drug of last resort to treat infections caused by bacteria already resistant to other drugs. Although the patient recovered, this case is still a cause for concern because the colistin-resistance gene, *mcr-1*, could spread to other bacteria.

May 2016   A study conducted by Tobin Hammer and colleagues at the University of Colorado finds that the dung of cattle that were administered tetracycline was dominated by drug-resistant microbes, while the microbes in cattle not given tetracycline harbored a more diverse colony of microbes that were not drug resistant.

June 2016   Research conducted at the University of Lisbon finds a rise in drug-resistant UTIs among household pets, including cats and dogs, raising the possibility that drug-resistant microbes could be transmitted to pets' human owners.

SOURCES FOR FURTHER INFORMATION

Adegbola, Richard A., and Debasish Saha. "Vaccines: A Cost-Effective Strategy to Contain Antimicrobial Resistance." In *Antimicrobial Resistance in Developing Countries,* edited by Annibal de J. Sosa, Denis K. Byarugaba, Carlos F. Amabile-Cuevas, Po-Ren Hsueh, Samuel Kariuki, and Iruka N. Okeke, 477–490. New York: Springer, 2010.

Agreja, Ashish, Naresh Bellam, and Susan R. Levy. "Strategies to Enhance Patient Adherence: Making It Simple." *MedGenMed* (2005) 7 (1): 4. http://www.ncbi .nlm.nih.gov/pmc/articles/PMC1681370 (accessed November 20, 2015)

American Chemical Society. "Selman Waksman and Antibiotics" (2005). http:// www.acs.org/content/acs/en/education/whatischemistry/landmarks /selmanwaksman.html (accessed April 29, 2015)

American College of Preventive Medicine. "Medication Adherence Clinical Reference" (2011). http://www.acpm.org/?MedAdherTT_ClinRef (accessed November 20, 2015)

American Veterinary Medical Association. Antimicrobial Use and Antimicrobial Resistance FAQ. https://www.avma.org/KB/Resources/FAQs/Pages/Antimi crobial-Use-and-Antimicrobial-Resistance-FAQs.aspx (accessed April 26, 2015)

Aminov, Rustam I. "A Brief History of the Antibiotic Era: Lessons Learned and Challenges for the Future." *Frontiers in Microbiology* 2010 (1): 134. http://journal.frontiersin.org/article/10.3389/fmicb.2010.00134/full (accessed April 26, 2015)

Bidgood, Jess, and Dave Phlipps. "Judge in Maine Eases Restrictions on Nurse." *The New York Times* (October 31, 2014). http://nyti.ms/1u0HcSh (accessed July 4, 2015)

Braine, Theresa. "Race Against Time to Develop New Antibiotics." *Bulletin of the World Health Organization* (2011) 89: 88–89. http://www.who.int/bulletin/ volumes/89/2/11-030211/en (accessed July 5, 2016)

Castanon, J. I. R. "History of the Use of Antibiotic as Growth Promoters in European Poultry Feeds." *Poultry Science* (2007) 86 (11): 2466–2471. http://ps.oxfordjournals.org/content/86/11/2466.long (accessed May 7, 2015)

Centers for Disease Control and Prevention (CDC). "About Antimicrobial Resistance" (September 16, 2013). http://www.cdc.gov/drugresistance/about.html (accessed April 26, 2015)

Centers for Disease Control and Prevention (CDC). "Antibiotic Resistance Threats in the United States, 2013." http://www.cdc.gov/drugresistance/pdf/ar-threats-2013-508.pdf (accessed April 26, 2015)

Centers for Disease Control and Prevention (CDC). "Antibiotic-Resistant Gonorrhea Basic Information." http://www.cdc.gov/std/gonorrhea/arg/basic.htm (accessed August 1, 2016)

Centers for Disease Control and Prevention (CDC). "Antibiotic Rx in Hospitals: Proceed with Caution." *Vital Signs* (March 2014). http://www.cdc.gov/vitalsigns/antibiotic-prescribing-practices (accessed September 4, 2015)

Centers for Disease Control and Prevention (CDC). "Core Elements of Hospital Antibiotic Stewardship Programs" (May 7, 2015). http://www.cdc.gov/getsmart/healthcare/implementation/core-elements.html (accessed May 16, 2015)

Centers for Disease Control and Prevention (CDC). "Ebola Guidance for Airlines" (October 15, 2014). http://www.cdc.gov/quarantine/air/managing-sick-travelers/ebola-guidance-airlines.html (accessed November 21, 2015)

Centers for Disease Control and Prevention (CDC). "Get Smart: When Antibiotics Work" (updated April 17, 2015). http://www.cdc.gov/getsmart/community/index.html (accessed September 1, 2015)

Centers for Disease Control and Prevention (CDC). "Gonorrhea—CDC Fact Sheet (Detailed Version)" (November 17, 2015). http://www.cdc.gov/std/gonorrhea/stdfact-gonorrhea-detailed.htm (accessed August 1, 2016)

Centers for Disease Control and Prevention (CDC). "Hospital-Associated Infections (HAIs)" (updated August 3, 2015). http://www.cdc.gov/HAI/prevent/prevention_tools.html (accessed September 1, 2015)

Centers for Disease Control and Prevention (CDC). "Improving Antibiotic Prescribing in Hospitals Can Make Health Care Safer." Press release (March 4, 2014). http://www.cdc.gov/media/releases/2014/p0304-poor-antibiotic-prescribing.html (accessed May 8, 2015)

Centers for Disease Control and Prevention (CDC). "Malaria." http://www.cdc.gov/malaria (accessed May 9, 2015)

Centers for Disease Control and Prevention (CDC). "Malaria Facts" (updated March 4, 2015). http://www.cdc.gov/malaria/about/facts.html (accessed May 4, 2015)

Centers for Disease Control and Prevention (CDC). *National and State Healthcare-Associated Infections: Progress Report* (2016). http://www.cdc.gov/HAI/pdfs/progress-report/hai-progress-report.pdf (accessed July 5, 2016)

Centers for Disease Control and Prevention (CDC). "Preventing Healthcare-Associated Infections" (November 16, 2015). http://www.cdc.gov/hai/prevent/prevention.html (accessed July 5, 2016)

Centers for Disease Control and Prevention (CDC). "Quarantine and Isolation" (October 22, 2015). http://www.cdc.gov/quarantine/index.html (accessed November 21, 2015)

Centers for Disease Control and Prevention (CDC). "Self-Study Modules on Tuberculosis: Patient Adherence to Tuberculosis Treatment" (October 1999). http://www.cdc.gov/tb/education/ssmodules/pdfs/9.pdf (accessed November 21, 2015)

Centers for Disease Control and Prevention (CDC). "Serotypes and the Importance of Serotyping Salmonella" (March 9, 2015). http://www.cdc.gov/salmonella/reportspubs/salmonella-atlas/serotyping-importance.html (accessed May 2, 2015)

Centers for Disease Control and Prevention (CDC). "Sexually Transmitted Disease Surveillance 2014" (November 2015). http://www.cdc.gov/std/stats14/surv-2014-print.pdf (accessed August 1, 2016)

Centers for Disease Control and Prevention (CDC). "Tuberculosis (TB)." http://www.cdc.gov/tb/default.htm (accessed May 8, 2015)

Christensen, Alan J. *Patient Adherence to Medical Treatment Regimens: Bridging the Gap Between Behavioral Science and Biomedicine*. New Haven: Yale University Press, 2004.

Cleveland Clinic. *Guidelines for Antimicrobial Usage: 2012–2013*. Cleveland: Cleveland Clinic, 2012. https://www.clevelandclinicmeded.com/medicalpubs/antimicrobial-guidelines/pdf/Antimicrobial-2013.pdf (accessed September 11, 2015)

Cogliani, Carol, Herman Goossens, and Christina Greko. "Restricting Antimicrobial Use in Food Animals: Lessons from Europe." *Microbe* (2011) 6 (6): 274–279. http://www.tufts.edu/med/apua/news/press_room_34_846139138.pdf (accessed May 7, 2015)

Daniel, Thomas M. "The History of Tuberculosis." *Respiratory Medicine* (November 2006) 100 (11): 1862–1870. http://www.sciencedirect.com/science/article/pii/S095461110600401X (accessed April 28, 2015)

de Craen, Anton J. M., Pieter J. Roos, A. Leonard de Vries, and Jos Kleijnen. "Effect of Colour of Drugs: Systematic Review of Perceived Effect of Drugs and their Effectiveness." *BMJ* 313 (December 1996), 21–28. http://www.ncbi.nlm.nih.gov/pmc/articles/PMC2359128/pdf/bmj00573-0060.pdf (accessed September 22, 2016)

De Groot, Maria J., and Katrien E. van't Hooft. "The Hidden Effects of Dairy Farming on Public and Environmental Health in the Netherlands, India, Ethiopia, and Uganda, Considering the Use of Antibiotics and Other Agro-Chemicals." *Frontiers in Public Health* (February 2016) 4 (12): 1–9. http://www.ncbi.nlm.nih.gov/pubmed/26942171 (accessed July 10, 2016)

De Vries, Theo P. G. M., R. H. Henning, H. V. Hogerzeil, and D. A. Fresle. *Guide to Good Prescribing: A Practical Manual*. Geneva, Switzerland: World Health Organization, 1994.

Drazen, Jeffrey M., Rupa Kanapathipillai, Edward W. Campion, Eric J. Rubin, Soctt M. Hammer, Stephen Morrisey, and Lindsey R. Baden. "Ebola and Quarantine." *New England Journal of Medicine* (November 20, 2014) 371 (21): 2029–2030.

European Center for Disease Control and Prevention (ECDC). "Antimicrobial Resistance: Factsheet for the General Public." http://ecdc.europa.eu/en /healthtopics/antimicrobial_resistance/basic_facts/Pages/factsheet_general _public.aspx (accessed April 26, 2015)

European Center for Disease Control and Prevention (ECDC). "Surveillance of Antimicrobial Consumption in Europe 2012." Stockholm: ECDC, 2014. http:// ecdc.europa.eu/en/publications/Publications/antimicrobial-consumption -europe-esac-net-2012.pdf (accessed April 28, 2015)

European Medicines Agency. "Sales of Veterinary Antimicrobial Agents in 26 EU/EEA Countries in 2013" (October 15, 2015). http://www.ema.europa.eu /docs/en_GB/document_library/Report/2015/10/WC500195687.pdf (accessed July 10, 2016)

Executive Office of the President, President's Council of Advisors on Science and Technology. "Report to the President on Combating Antibiotic Resistance" (September 2014). https://www.whitehouse.gov/sites/default/files/microsites /ostp/PCAST/pcast_carb_report_sept2014.pdf (accessed September 7, 2015)

Fink, Sheri. "Ebola Crisis Passes, but Questions on Quarantines Persist." *The New York Times* (December 2, 2015). http://nyti.ms/1LPpfJy (accessed July 4, 2015)

Food and Agriculture Organization of the United Nations (FAO). "Animal Production and Health." http://www.fao.org/ag/againfo/themes/en/Environment .html (accessed July 10, 2016)

Food and Agriculture Organization of the United Nations (FAO). "Antibiotics in Farm Animal Production: Public Health and Animal Welfare." http://www.fao .org/fileadmin/user_upload/animalwelfare/antibiotics_in_animal_farming .pdf (accessed July 10, 2016)

Frith, John. "Syphilis—Its Early History and Treatment Until Penicillin and the Debate on Its Origin." *Journal of Military and Veterans Health* (November 2012) 20 (4): 49–58. http://jmvh.org/wp-content/uploads/2013/03/Frith .pdf (accessed April 29, 2015)

Gellard, W.F., J. L. Grenard, and Z. A. Marcum. "A Systematic Review of Barriers to Medication Adherence in the Elderly: Looking Beyond Cost and Regime Complexity." *American Journal of Geriatric Pharmacotherapy* (February 2011) 9(1): 11–23. http://www.ncbi.nlm.nih.gov/pmc/articles/PMC308 4587 (accessed November 20, 2015)

Haak, Hilbrand, and Aryanti Radyowijati. "Determinants of Antimicrobial Use: Poorly Understood—Poorly Researched." In *Antimicrobial Resistance in*

Developing Countries, edited by Annibal de J. Sosa, Denis K. Byarugaba, Carlos F. Amabile-Cuevas, Po-Ren Hsueh, Samuel Kariuki, and Iruka N. Okeke, 283–300. New York: Springer, 2010.

Harvard School of Public Health. "Obesity Prevention Source: Food and Diet." https://www.hsph.harvard.edu/obesity-prevention-source/obesity-causes/diet-and-weight (accessed July 10, 2016)

Hughes, Peter, and John Heritage. "Antibiotic Growth-Promoters in Food Animals." In *Assessing Quality and Safety of Animal Feeds,* 129–152. Rome: Food and Agriculture Organization of the United Nations, 2004. http://www.fao.org/docrep/article/agrippa/555_en.htm (accessed May 7, 2015)

Hunink, M. G. Myriam, and Paul P. Glasziou. *Decision Making in Health and Medicine: Integrating Evidence and Values.* Cambridge, UK: Cambridge University Press, 2011.

Innovative Medicines Initiative. http://www.imi.europa.eu (accessed September 7, 2015)

IOM Forum on Microbial Threats. *Infectious Disease Movement in a Borderless World: Workshop Summary.* "Globalization, Movement of Pathogens (and Their Hosts), and the Revised International Health Regulations," December 16–17, 2008. Washington, DC: National Academies Press, 2010. https://www.nap.edu/read/12758/chapter/1 (accessed September 22, 2016)

Jin, Jing, Grant Edward Sklar, Vernon Min She Oh, and Shu Chuen Li. "Factors Affecting Therapeutic Compliance: A Review from the Patient's Perspective." *Therapeutics and Clinical Risk Management* 2008:4 (1): 269–286.

Kristiansson, Erik, Jerker Fick, Anders Janzon, Roman Grabic, Carolin Rutgersson, Birgitta Weijdegård, Hanna Söderström, and D. G. Joakim Larsson. "Pyrosequencing of Antibiotic-Contaminated River Sediments Reveals High Levels of Resistance and Gene Transfer Elements." *PLOS One* (February 2011) 6 (2). http://www.plosone.org/article/fetchObject.action?uri=info:doi/10.1371/journal.pone.0017038&representation=PDF (accessed September 3, 2015)

Lax, Eric. *The Mold in Dr. Florey's Coat: The Story of the Penicillin Miracle.* New York: Henry Holt, 2004.

Lee, Grace C., Kelly R. Reveles, Russell T. Attridge, Kenneth A. Lawson, Ishak A. Mansi, James S. Lewis, and Christopher R. Frei. "Outpatient Antibiotic Prescribing in the United States: 2000 to 2010." *BMC Medicine* (June 11, 2014) 12: 96. http://www.biomedcentral.com/1741-7015/12/96 (accessed September 1, 2015)

Lesch, John E. *The First Miracle Drugs: How the Sulfa Drugs Transformed Medicine.* New York: Oxford University Press, 2007.

Levy, Stuart B., G. B. Fitzgerald, and A. B. Macone. "Spread of Antibiotic Resistance Plasmids from Chicken to Chicken and from Chicken to Man." *Nature* (1976) 260: 40–42.

Llor, Carl, Silvia Hernandez, Carolina Bayona, Ana Moragas, Nuria Sierra, Marta Hernandez, and Marc Miravitlles. "A Study of Adherence to Antibiotic Treatment in Ambulatory Respiratory Infections." *International Journal of Infectious*

Diseases (2013) 17: e168–e172. http://www.ijidonline.com/article/S1201-9712 (12)01265-9/pdf (accessed November 20, 2015)

Mackowiak, Philip A., and Paul S. Sehdev. "The Origin of Quarantine." *Clinical Infectious Diseases* (2002) 35 (9): 1071–1072. http://cid.oxfordjournals.org /content/35/9/1071.long (accessed July 4, 2016)

Mainous, Arch G., Charles J. Everett, Robert E. Post, Vanessa A. Diaz, and William J. Hueston. "Availability of Antibiotics for Purchase Without a Prescription on the Internet." *Annals of Family Medicine* (September/October 2009) 7 (5): 431–435. http://www.ncbi.nlm.nih.gov/pmc/articles/PMC2746509/pdf /0060431.pdf (accessed May 8, 2015)

Markel, Howard. "The Real Story Behind Penicillin." *PBS Newshour* (September 27, 2013). http://www.pbs.org/newshour/rundown/the-real-story-behind -the-worlds-first-antibiotic (accessed April 28, 2015)

Moyer, Justin William. "Kaci Hickox, Rebel Ebola Nurse Loathed by Conservatives, Sues Chris Christie over Quarantine." *Washington Post* (October 23, 2015). https://www.washingtonpost.com/news/morning-mix/wp/2015/10/23 /kaci-hickox-rebel-ebola-nurse-loathed-by-conservatives-sues-chris-christie -over-quarantine (accessed July 5, 2015)

Nalule, Yolisa. "Is Physician Education Effective in Promoting Antibiotic Stewardship?" *Policy Brief 11* (February 2011). New York: The Center for Disease Dynamics, Economics, and Policy, 2011. http://www.shea-online.org/Portals /0/Policy_Brief_11.pdf (accessed September 11, 2015)

National Health Service (NHS). "Antibiotics" (reviewed May 6, 2014). http://www .nhs.uk/conditions/Antibiotics-penicillins/Pages/Introduction.aspx (accessed April 28, 2015)

National Institute of Allergy and Infectious Diseases. "E. coli." http://www.niaid .nih.gov/topics/ecoli/understanding/pages/cause.aspx (accessed April 29, 2015)

National Institute of Allergy and Infectious Diseases. "Flu (Influenza)." http://www .niaid.nih.gov/topics/flu/Pages/default.aspx (accessed May 9, 2015)

National Pesticide Information Center, Oregon State University. "Antimicrobials: Topic Fact Sheet." http://npic.orst.edu/factsheets/antimicrobials.html (accessed April 27, 2015)

Nicolle, Lindsay E. *Infection Control Programmes to Control Antimicrobial Resistance.* Geneva, Switzerland: World Health Organization, 2001. http://apps .who.int/iris/bitstream/10665/66859/1/WHO_CDS_CSR_DRS_2001.7.pdf (accessed September 1, 2015)

Nieuwlaat, R., N. Wilczynski, T. Navarro, N. Hobson, R. Jeffery, A. Keepanasseril, T. Agoritsas, et al. "Interventions for Enhancing Medication Adherence." *Cochrane Database Systematic Reviews.* http://onlinelibrary.wiley.com/doi/10 .1002/14651858.CD000011.pub4/abstract;jsessionid=8EEA718C8E215A40 060E5B0BBE36A11B.f01t03 (accessed November 20, 2014)

Okeke, Iruka N. "Poverty and Root Causes of Resistance in Developing Countries." In *Antimicrobial Resistance in Developing Countries,* edited by Annibal de J.

Sosa, Denis K. Byarugaba, Carlos F. Amabile-Cuevas, Po-Ren Hsueh, Samuel Kariuki, and Iruka N. Okeke, 27–36. New York: Springer, 2010. http://www .tufts.edu/med/apua/about_us/publications_21_3125925763.pdf (accessed May 8, 2015)

O'Neill, Jim, and the Review on Antimicrobial Resistance. "Antimicrobials in Agriculture and the Environment: Reducing Unnecessary Use and Waste." (December 2015). http://amr-review.org/sites/default/files/Antimicrobials%20 in%20agriculture%20and%20the%20environment%20-%20Reducing%20 unnecessary%20use%20and%20waste.pdf (accessed July 10, 2016)

O'Neill, Jim, and the Review on Antimicrobial Resistance. "Infection Prevention, Control, and Surveillance: Limiting the Development and Spread of Drug Resistance" (March 2016). http://amr-review.org/sites/default/files/Health%20 infrastructure%20and%20surveillance%20final%20version_LR_NO%20 CROPS.pdf (accessed July 5, 2016)

O'Neill, Jim, and the Review on Antimicrobial Resistance. "Securing New Drugs for Future Generations: The Pipeline of Antibiotics" (May 2015). http://amr -review.org/sites/default/files/SECURING%20NEW%20DRUGS%20 FOR%20FUTURE%20GENERATIONS%20FINAL%20WEB_0.pdf (accessed July 5, 2016)

Ozawa, Sachiko, Meghan L. Stack, David M. Bishai, Andrew Mirelman, Ingrid K. Friberg, Louis Niessen, Damian G. Walker, and Orin S. Levine. "During the 'Decade of Vaccines,' The Lives of 6.4 Million Children Valued at $231 Billion Could Be Saved." *Health Affairs* (June 2011) 30 (6): 1010–1020. http://content .healthaffairs.org/content/30/6/1010.full?ijkey=aCQyO70nhG4zw&keytype =ref&siteid=healthaff (accessed September 1, 2015)

Packard, Randall M. "The Origins of Antimalarial-Drug Resistance." *New England Journal of Medicine* (July 31, 2014) 371 (5): 397–399.

Pew Charitable Trusts. "Antibiotics Currently in Clinical Development" (July 2015). http://www.pewtrusts.org/~/media/assets/2015/03/antibioticsinnovationpro ject_datatable_march2015.pdf?la=en (accessed July 5, 2016)

Pew Charitable Trusts. "From Lab Bench to Bedside: A Backgrounder on Drug Development" (March 12, 2014). http://www.pewtrusts.org/en/about/news -room/news/2014/03/12/from-lab-bench-to-bedside-a-backgrounder-on -drug-development (accessed September 7, 2015)

Pew Charitable Trusts. "Tracking the Pipeline of Antibiotics in Development." (March 12, 2014, updated May 2016). http://www.pewtrusts.org/en/research -and-analysis/issue-briefs/2014/03/12/tracking-the-pipeline-of-antibiotics-in -development (accessed July 5, 2016)

Phillips, Patrick J., Steven G. Smith, D. W. Kolpin, Steven D. Zaugg, Herbert T. Buxton, Edward T. Furlong, Kathleen Esposito, and Beverley Stinson. "Pharmaceutical Formulation Facilities as Sources of Opioids and Other Pharmaceuticals to Wastewater Treatment Plant Effluents." *Environmental Science and Technology* (2010) 44: 4910–4916. http://pubs.acs.org/doi/ipdf/10.1021 /es100356f (accessed September 3, 2015)

Rosenblatt-Farrell, Noah. "The Landscape of Antibiotic Resistance." *Environmental Health Perspectives* (June 2009) 117 (6): A244–A250. http://www.ncbi .nlm.nih.gov/pmc/articles/PMC2702430 (accessed April 28, 2015)

Stack, Meghan L., Sachiko Ozawa, David M. Bishai, Andrew Mirelman, Yvonne Tam, Louis Niessen, Damian G. Walker, and Orin S. Levine. "Estimated Economic Benefits During the 'Decade of Vaccines' Include Treatment Savings, Gains in Labor Productivity." *Health Affairs* (June 2011) 30 (6): 1021–1028. http://content.healthaffairs.org/content/30/6/1021.full?ijkey=2aMaZBnn JqWz6&keytype=ref&siteid=healthaff (accessed September 1, 2015)

Sukkar, Elizabeth. "Why Are There So Few Antibiotics in the Research and Development Pipeline?" *The Pharmaceutical Journal* (November 2013). http:// www.pharmaceutical-journal.com/news-and-analysis/features/why-are-there -so-few-antibiotics-in-the-research-and-development-pipeline/11130209 .article (accessed September 7, 2015)

Todar, Kenneth. *Todar's Online Textbook of Bacteriology*. http://textbookofbac teriology.net/index.html (accessed April 26, 2015)

Tyson, Peter. "A Short History of Quarantine" (October 12, 2004). http://www.pbs .org/wgbh/nova/body/short-history-of-quarantine.html (accessed November 21, 2015)

U.S. Department of Agriculture. Dietary Guidelines for Americans 2015–2020. 8th ed. http://health.gov/dietaryguidelines/2015/resources/2015-2020_Die tary_Guidelines.pdf (accessed July 10, 2016)

U.S. Department of Health and Human Services. "HIV/AIDS 101: Global Statistics." https://www.aids.gov/hiv-aids-basics/hiv-aids-101/global-statistics/index .html (accessed May 9, 2015)

U.S. Department of Health and Human Services. "HIV/AIDS 101: U.S. Statistics." https://www.aids.gov/hiv-aids-basics/hiv-aids-101/statistics (accessed May 9, 2015)

U.S. Department of Health and Human Services. "Overview of HIV Treatments." https://www.aids.gov/hiv-aids-basics/just-diagnosed-with-hiv-aids/treatment -options/overview-of-hiv-treatments (accessed May 9, 2015)

U.S. Food and Drug Administration (FDA). 2013 Summary Report on Antimicrobials Sold or Distributed for Use in Food-Producing Animals (April 2015). http://www.fda.gov/downloads/ForIndustry/UserFees/AnimalDrugUserFee ActADUFA/UCM440584.pdf (accessed July 10, 2016)

U.S. Food and Drug Administration (FDA). "The Drug Development Process." (June 24, 2015). http://www.fda.gov/ForPatients/Approvals/Drugs/default.htm (accessed July 5, 2016)

U.S. Food and Drug Administration (FDA). "FDA's Strategy on Antimicrobial Resistance—Questions and Answers." http://www.fda.gov/AnimalVeterinary /GuidanceComplianceEnforcement/GuidanceforIndustry/ucm216939.htm (accessed July 10, 2016)

U.S. Food and Drug Administration (FDA). "How Does FDA Decide When a Drug Is not Safe Enough to Stay on the Market?" (May 12, 2016). http://www.fda .gov/AboutFDA/Transparency/Basics/ucm194984.htm (accessed July 5, 2016)

U.S. Food and Drug Administration (FDA). "The National Antimicrobial Resistance Monitoring System." http://www.fda.gov/AnimalVeterinary/Safety Health/AntimicrobialResistance/NationalAntimicrobialResistanceMonitoring System/default.htm (accessed July 10, 2016)

Van Boeckel, Thomas P., Sumanth Gandra, Ashvin Ashok, Quentin Caudron, Bryan T. Grenfell, Simon A. Levin, and Ramanan Laxminarayan. "Antibiotic Consumption 2000 to 2010: An Analysis of National Pharmaceutical Sales Data." *The Lancet: Infectious Diseases* (August 2014) 14 (8): 742–750. https:// www.princeton.edu/~slevin/PDF/Levinpubs/PDFWEB2014/515_VanBoec kelGlobal_2014.pdf (accessed April 28, 2015).

World Health Organization (WHO). *Adherence to Long-Term Therapies: Evidence for Action.* Geneva, Switzerland: World Health Organization, 2003. http://apps.who.int/iris/bitstream/10665/42682/1/9241545992.pdf (accessed November 20, 2015)

World Health Organization (WHO). "Antimicrobial Resistance." Fact Sheet No. 194 (updated April 2014). http://www.who.int/mediacentre/factsheets/ fs194/en (accessed April 26, 2015)

World Health Organization (WHO). *Antimicrobial Resistance: Global Report on Surveillance 2014.* Geneva, Switzerland: World Health Organization, 2015. http://www.who.int/drugresistance/documents/surveillancereport/en (accessed May 2, 2015)

World Health Organization (WHO). "Antimicrobial Resistance." Sixty-seventh World Health Assembly, Agenda Item 16.5. May 24, 2014. http://apps.who .int/gb/ebwha/pdf_files/WHA67/A67_R25-en.pdf?ua=1&ua=1 (accessed September 4, 2015)

World Health Organization (WHO). "Drug Resistance: Global Strategy Recommendations: Physicians and Dispensers." http://www.who.int/drugresistance/ WHO_Global_Strategy_Recommendations/en/index1.html (accessed September 11, 2015)

World Health Organization (WHO). "Emergence of Multi-drug Resistant *Neisseria gonorrhoeae*—Threat of Global Rise in Untreatable Sexually Transmitted Infections" (2011). http://whqlibdoc.who.int/hq/2011/WHO_RHR_11.14 _eng.pdf?ua=1 (accessed May 2, 2015)

World Health Organization (WHO). "Global Incidence and Prevalence of Selected Curable Sexually Transmitted Infections—2008." http://www.who .int/reproductivehealth/publications/rtis/stisestimates/en (accessed August 1, 2016)

World Health Organization (WHO). *Global Tuberculosis Report 2015.* 20th ed. Geneva, Switzerland: World Health Organization, 2015. http://apps.who.int /iris/bitstream/10665/191102/1/9789241565059_eng.pdf?ua=1 (accessed November 21, 2015)

World Health Organization (WHO). *Guidelines for the Treatment of Malaria.* 3rd ed. Geneva, Switzerland: World Health Organization, 2015. http://apps .who.int/iris/bitstream/10665/162441/1/9789241549127_eng.pdf?ua=1 (accessed May 9, 2015)

World Health Organization (WHO). "Infection Control Standard Precautions in Health Care" (2006). http://www.who.int/csr/resources/publications/4EPR_AM2.pdf (accessed July 5, 2016)

World Health Organization (WHO). "The Medical Impact of Antimicrobial Use in Food Animals. Report of a WHO Meeting. Berlin, Germany, 13–17 October 1997." WHO/EMC/ZOO/97.4. http://apps.who.int/iris/bitstream/10665/64439/1/WHO_EMC_ZOO_97.4.pdf (accessed September 23, 2016)

World Health Organization (WHO). "Public Health Surveillance" (2016). http://www.who.int/topics/public_health_surveillance/en (accessed July 6, 2016)

World Health Organization (WHO). "Pursue High-Quality DOTS Expansion and Enhancement" (2015). http://www.who.int/tb/dots/en (accessed November 21, 2015)

World Health Organization (WHO). "Q & A on Artemisinin Resistance" (February 2015). http://www.who.int/malaria/media/artemisinin_resistance_qa/en (accessed May 9, 2015)

World Health Organization (WHO). "Race Against Time to Develop New Antibiotics." *Bulletin of the World Health Organization* (2011) 29: 88–89. http://www.who.int/bulletin/volumes/89/2/11-030211/en (accessed May 14, 2015)

World Health Organization (WHO). Sexually Transmitted Infections (STIs). Fact Sheet No. 110 (December 2015). http://www.who.int/mediacentre/factsheets/fs110/en (accessed August 1, 2016)

World Health Organization (WHO). "Tuberculosis (TB)." http://www.who.int/topics/tuberculosis/en (accessed May 8, 2015)

World Health Organization (WHO). "WHO Guidance on Human Rights and Involuntary Detention for XDR-TB Control" (January 24, 2007). http://www.who.int/tb/features_archive/involuntary_treatment/en (accessed November 21, 2015)

World Health Organization (WHO). *WHO Guidelines for the Treatment of* Neisseria gonorrhoeae. Geneva, Switzerland: World Health Organization, 2016. http://apps.who.int/iris/bitstream/10665/246114/1/9789241549691-eng.pdf?ua=1 (accessed August 1, 2016)

World Health Organization (WHO). *WHO Model List of Essential Medicines.* 18th ed. (Revised October 2013). http://apps.who.int/iris/bitstream/10665/93142/1/EML_18_eng.pdf?ua=1 (accessed April 28, 2015)

World Health Organization (WHO). "World Health Day 2011: Policy Package to Combat Antimicrobial Resistance." http://www.who.int/world-health-day/2011/presskit/WHDIntrototobriefs.pdf?ua=1 (accessed May 8, 2015)

World Health Organization (WHO). *World Malaria Report 2015.* Geneva, Switzerland: World Health Organization, 2015. http://apps.who.int/iris/bitstream/10665/200018/1/9789241565158_eng.pdf (accessed September 22, 2016).

World Health Organization (WHO). *The World Medicines Situation: 2011.* Geneva, Switzerland: World Health Organization, forthcoming (some chapters available

2016. http://apps.who.int/medicinedocs/documents/s20054en/s20054en.pdf ?ua=1 (accessed Sept 22, 2016)

World Health Organization (WHO). *Worldwide Country Situation Analysis: Response to Antimicrobial Resistance.* Geneva, Switzerland: World Health Organization, 2015. http://apps.who.int/iris/bitstream/10665/163468/1/978 9241564946_eng.pdf?ua=1 (accessed May 8, 2015)

GLOSSARY

***Acinetobacter baumannii*:** A species of aerobic, Gram-negative bacteria resistant to most antibiotics. *A. baumannii* can cause disease in humans, including pneumonia, urinary tract infections (UTIs), and bloodstream infections.

Aminoglysides: A class of antibiotics, including gentamicin and amikacin, that bind to ribosomal subunits and interfere with protein synthesis in bacteria.

Antibiogram: An *in vitro* test to determine the sensitivity of a strain of bacteria to different antibiotics.

Antibiotics: Also called *antibacterials*, antibiotics are drugs that are able to kill or otherwise interfere with the normal processes of bacteria. There are many broad classes of antibiotics, including the penicillins, the sulfanomides, and the tetracyclines.

Antifungals: Drugs that are able to kill or otherwise interfere with the normal processes of fungi. Examples of antifungal drugs include clotrimazole, miconazole, and amphotericin.

Antimicrobials: Any drugs or other agents that interfere with the normal growth or function of any microscopic organism, such as bacteria or viruses. Many antimicrobials kill organisms, but others may act against them by other means, such as preventing them from reproducing. The term *antimicrobial* is a broad category that includes many different types of drugs and other agents, such as antibiotics (which are effective against bacteria) and antivirals (which are effective against viruses).

Antiparasitics: Drugs that are able to kill or otherwise interfere with the normal processes of parasites. Examples of antiparasitic drugs include rifampin, tinizadole, and niclosamide.

Beta-lactam antibiotics: Also writtens as *β-lactam antibiotics*, a widely used class of antibiotics that includes carbapenems, cephalosporins, monobactams, and penams (penicillin derivatives).

Biomedical Advanced Research and Development Authority (BARDA): An authority within the U.S. Department of Health and Human Services. Its purpose is to provide a systematic and integrated approach to the development and purchase of items needed to respond to public health emergencies, including drugs, diagnostic tools, and vaccines.

Brand name: Also called a *trade name*, a name assigned to a drug marketed by a specific manufacturer. For instance, Azithromax and AzaSite are brand names for drugs whose active ingredient is the antibiotic azithromycin.

Broad-spectrum antibiotics: Antibiotics that are effective against many types of bacteria. An example of a broad-spectrum antibiotic is ampicillin, which is effective against both Gram-positive and Gram-negative types of bacteria, including some types of *Streptococcus, Enterococci,* and *Enterobacteriaceae.* One advantage of broad-spectrum antibiotics is that they may be effective in treating illness even if the specific type of bacteria causing the illness is not known.

Cephalosporins: A class of beta-lactam antibiotics derived from *Acremonium*; they are effective against some types of both Gram-negative and Gram-positive bacteria.

Commensals: Organisms that exist in a mutually symbiotic relationship but are not entirely dependent on each other; one example is the gut microbiome.

Conjugation: One process through which cells can exchange genetic materials, which is one method by which antibiotic resistance can be exchanged from one cell to another.

Enteric bacteria: Bacteria that live in the intestines of living beings, such as humans or cattle.

***Enterobacter*:** A common genus of Gram-negative bacteria, some of which cause illness in humans. Persons with compromised immune systems and those being treated by mechanical ventilation are most vulnerable, with the most common infection sites being the respiratory and urinary tracts.

Extremely drug-resistant tuberculosis (XDR TB): A disease caused by infection with a strain of the bacteria *Mycobacterium tuberculosis* that is resistant not only to isoniazid and rifampim, two drugs commonly used to treat TB, but also to most of the alternative drugs available to treat the disease.

First-line drugs: Drugs most commonly used to treat an illness. If the first-line drugs are not effective (for instance, if an infection is caused by a type of bacteria resistant to these drugs), then second-line drugs may be employed to treat the infection. For instance, when treating tuberculosis (TB), first-line drugs include the antibiotics isoniazid and rifampin, while second-line drugs include the fluoroquinolones.

Fungicide: An organism or chemical compound that can kill or inhibit the growth of fungal spores or fungi.

Fungus: A type of organism that has multiple cells with nuclei and cell walls but does not contain chlorophyll. Some fungi cause diseases in humans, animals, or plants, but not all are harmful. For instance, yeast is nutritious and is used in making bread and beer, and penicillin, an important antibiotic, also comes from a fungus.

Generic drug name: A generic drug name gives the name of the active ingredient in a drug, rather than a name given by a specific manufacturer. For instance, azithromycin is the generic name of an antibiotic of the macrolide class; the brand or trade names for drugs whose active ingredient is azithromycin include Zithromax and AzaSite.

Genes: Units of heredity composed of a segment of a deoxyribonucleic acid (DNA) molecule. They carry the instructions for creating proteins and are a means for inherited characteristics to be passed from generation to generation.

Gene transfer: One of the ways that microbes develop antimicrobial resistance, in which a gene conferring a quality such as antimicrobial resistance is passed from one microorganism to another, with the receiving microorganism thus acquiring the property coded in the gene.

Gram-negative bacteria: Following the Gram-staining procedure, Gram-positive bacteria are stained pink. Gram-negative bacteria have a thin peptidoglycan layer (a polymer of amino acids and sugars) and an outer layer that Gram-positive bacteria do not have, which is made up of lipids, proteins, and polysaccharides. Examples of Gram-negative bacteria include *Escherichia coli*, *Klebsiella pneumoniae*, and *Neisseria gonorrhoeae*.

Gram-positive bacteria: Following the Gram-staining procedure, Gram-positive bacteria are stained purple. Gram-positive bacteria have a thick peptidoglycan layer (a polymer of amino acids and sugars) that retains the crystal violet stain used in the first stage of the Gram-staining process. Gram-positive bacteria also lack the outer layer of lipids, proteins, and polysaccharides that Gram-negative bacteria have. Examples of Gram-positive bacteria include the *Streptococcus* and *Staphylococcus* types.

Gram staining: A method of identifying bacteria that was developed in the 19th century by the Danish bacteriologist Hans Christian Joachim Gram. Gram staining is a multistage lab process that subjects bacteria to two different dyes: crystal violet (the primary stain) and safranin (the counterstain). At the end of the procedure, Gram-positive bacteria are stained purple, and Gram-negative bacteria are stained pink.

Growth promoters: Chemicals used to stimulate growth in agricultural animals such as cattle. Low doses of antibiotics are sometimes used as growth promoters, but this practice has been criticized because it can lead to the development of antibiotic-resistant bacteria that also can infect humans.

Herpes simplex: The virus that causes genital herpes; it can be treated with acyclovir.

Horizontal gene transfer: Any of a number of processes by which an organism can receive genetic material from another organism without the first organism being the offspring of the second.

Immunoglobulins: A class of proteins that function as antibiotics; they are produced in the lymph tissues of vertebrates.

Integron: An element of DNA that can capture and carry genes by site-specific recombination; these are mobile elements that can promote antibiotic resistance.

Intrinsic resistance genes: Genes that do not specifically carry the code for the trait of antibiotic resistance but have the code for traits that may reduce sensitivity to antibiotics.

Macrolides: A family of antibiotics that bind to the large unit of a bacterial ribosome and thus inhibit protein synthesis. Examples include azithromycin, clindamysin, and erythromycin.

Methicillin-resistant *Staphylococcus aureus* (MRSA): A type of *Staphylococcus* (staph) that has been observed in both hospital and community settings and can cause serious illness in humans. Severe infections caused by MRSA are often treated with intravenous vancomycin, while less serious infections (e.g., boils on the skin) may be treated by incision and draining.

Multidrug-resistant tuberculosis (MDR TB): A disease caused by infection with drug-resistant strains of the bacteria *Mycobacterium tuberculosis*. MDR TB is resistant to at least two of the drugs commonly used to treat TB, isoniazid and rifampim, and patients with MDR TB may require at least two years of treatment with several different drugs before they are cured.

Multiple drug–resistant (MDR) bacteria: Bacteria that are resistant to several classes of antibiotics. The development of MDR strains of bacteria is a concern because they reduce the options available to medical science to treat infections caused by these bacteria. In the worst cases, there may be no effective treatment available, while in other cases, the treatments may be more expensive or have more side effects than the treatments used with non-MDR bacteria.

Mutation: One of the ways that microbes become resistant to antimicrobials. This is a random process, but because most microbes divide quickly (for instance, every few hours), the probability of mutations creating antimicrobial resistance is good. Due to selective pressure, those microbes with mutations that give them antimicrobial resistance are able to survive and reproduce, thus coming to represent a larger share of the population of microbes.

Narrow-spectrum antibiotics: Antibiotics effective against only a specific bacteria or specific group of bacterial types. The effective use of narrow-spectrum antibiotics requires that the type of bacteria causing an illness be known, so the correct antibiotic is chosen.

Necrotizing fasciitis: A skin infection that can be caused by a number of bacteria, including types of *Streptococcus* and *Staphyloccus*; because it can progress rapidly and infects deep layers of skin and subcutaneous tissue, it is sometimes called "flesh-eating disease."

Neisseria gonorrhoeae: The pathogen that causes gonorrhea, a sexually transmitted disease. Some strains of gonorrhea are resistant to most drugs, while others can be treated with antibiotics such as ceftriaxone or azithromycin.

Noninferiority trial: A clinical trial designed to demonstrate that a particular drug or treatment is as effective as (i.e., not inferior to) a currently existing drug.

This is a different approach from most clinical trials, which are designed to demonstrate that one drug or treatment is superior to others.

Nosocomial infection: An infection acquired while receiving treatment in a hospital. Sometimes the term *nosocomial* is used to describe an infection acquired in any healthcare facility, such as a medical clinic or long-term care facility.

Pathogen: A substance that can cause disease.

Pelvic inflammatory disease (PID): A condition that can be caused by infection with a number of different pathogens, including *Chlamydia trachomatis, Neisseria gonorrhoeae, Streptococci, Enterobacteriaceae,* and *Mycoplasma hominis.*

Penicillins: A class of beta-lactam antibiotics derived from the *Penicillium* fungi, used primarily to treat diseases caused by Gram-positive bacteria; historically, penicillins constituted the first class of antibiotic effective in treating many serious diseases.

Persister cells: Within a bacterial population, dormant cells that are highly resistant to antibiotics.

Phage therapy: Also called *bacteriophage therapy,* the use of viruses to combat bacterial infections. The potential of phage therapy was discovered in the early 20th century, but was largely left undeveloped in favor of antibiotic use except in the Soviet Union. However, in recent years, increasing antibiotic resistance has rekindled interest in phage therapy.

Plasmid: A piece of genetic material that is not part of a chromosome and can be transferred between bacteria (such transfer is one means by which antibiotic resistance can be passed among bacteria).

Polypeptide antibiotics: A class of antibiotics, including actinomycin, bacitracin, and polymixin B, that are used to treat infections of the bladder, ear, and eye. They are usually administered through inhalation or application to the eye or skin rather than systematically, due to their toxicity.

Pseudomonas aeruginosa: A bacterium found in most artificial environments, as well as in skin flora, soil, and water. Infection with *P. aeruginosa* causes inflammation and can be fatal if it occurs in organs such as the kidneys or lungs.

Quinolones: A class of synthetic antibiotics, including ciprofloxacin and fluoroquinolone, that inhibit bacterial replication.

Resistome: All genes that create antibiotic resistance, whether indirectly or directly.

Second-line drugs: Drugs used to treat an illness when the more common treatments, called *first-line drugs,* are not effective against it. For instance, first-line drugs used to treat tuberculosis (TB) include the antibiotics isoniazid and rifampin. If neither drug is effective, the infection is classified as multidrug-resistant TB (MDR TB), and second-line drugs such as the fluoroquinolones may be tried against the infection.

Selective pressure: A natural process that helps create antimicrobial resistance. When a colony of microbes is exposed to an antimicrobial, those microbes that are vulnerable to the antimicrobial will be killed, while those that are resistant will survive and be able to reproduce themselves. Over time, this process favors the development of antimicrobial resistance because the resistant microbes are able to survive and reproduce, so they will come to represent a greater fraction of the population of a particular type of microbe, while the vulnerable microbes of this type will be killed and thus cannot reproduce.

***Staphylococcus aureus*:** A Gram-positive bacteria commonly found on the skin and nose, which is a common cause of staph infections.

Subtherapeutic dose: An amount of a drug that is not sufficient to cure or prevent disease. One common use of subtherapeutic doses of antibiotics is the inclusion of small amounts of antibiotics in animal feed because this use of antibiotics has been shown to promote animal growth. One danger in the use of subtherapeutic doses of antibiotics is that this practice can promote the development of resistant strains of bacteria, which also may infect humans.

Superbug: A colloquial term for bacteria that have become resistant to many types of antibiotics. These bacteria pose a serious health hazard because infections caused by them are often difficult to treat effectively. Examples of superbugs include strains of *Staphylocuccus aureus* resistant to both methicillin and vancomycin (and many other types of antibiotics), and multidrug-resistant *Mycobacterium tuberculosis*, which causes multidrug-resistant tuberculosis (MDR TB).

Superinfection: A secondary infection; i.e., an infection that occurs when a patient is being treated for a different infection.

Tetracyclines: A class of antibiotics that are often used to treat patients allergic to the beta-lactams and macrolides. They act by inhibiting protein synthesis and are used to treat gonorrhea and infections of the urinary tract, intestines, sinuses, middle ear, and respiratory tract.

***Treponema pallidum*:** The bacteria that causes syphilis; it is usually treated with penicillin or doxycycline.

Vancomycin-resistant *Enterococci* (VCE): A type of *Enterococcus* bacteria that is resistant to vancomycin, as well as other types of antibiotics. *Enterococcus* bacteria commonly live in the human digestive tract and female genital tract and do not normally cause illness. However, they can cause serious infections in other parts of the body. Infection with VCE most commonly occurs in healthcare settings, where patients may have weakened immune systems and undergo invasive procedures that allow the bacteria to get into parts of the body where they can cause illness, such as the bloodstream.

Viruses: Infective agents consisting of a strand of genetic material [either ribonucleic acid (RNA) or deoxyribonucleic acid (DNA)] and a protein coat. They are extremely small compared to bacteria, and they can only reproduce into the cells of a host. Viruses are not vulnerable to antibiotics, but they are vulnerable to antiviral agents. Examples of diseases caused by viruses include the common cold and acquired immune deficiency syndrome (AIDS).

Index

Acinetobacter, 37
Acute otitis media (AOM), middle ear infection, 62–63
Animal husbandry, antibiotic use in, 24, 127–138; scope of antibiotic use in Europe, 133–134; scope of antibiotic use in United States, 132–133
Animal-to-human transmission of antibiotic-resistant pathogens, 128–129
Antibiotic manufacturing and water pollution, 81
Antibiotics: classes of, 5; consumption in Europe, 13, 20–21; global sales, 12–13; inappropriate use of, 19–20
Antimicrobial folk culture in developing countries, 65
Antimicrobial resistance: defined, 13–14; global overview of, 25–33; health and economic burden of, 33–34; mechanisms producing, 15–16; multidrug resistance, 14; reasons for concern, 16–17; United States overview of, 34, 42

Antiseptics in surgery, 7–8
Arsphenamine (Salversan), 8–9
Artemisinin, 32; resistance in Greater Mekong subregion, 50–51
Artemisinin-based combination therapy (ACT), 32

Bacteria: gram-negative and gram-positive, 6–7
Bacteriostasis, 11
Beta-lactams (β-lactams), 6
Biomedical Advanced Research and Development Authority (BARDA), U.S. Dept. of Health and Human Services, 92
Broad-spectrum antimicrobials, 3
Bronchiolitis, 63–64
Bronchitis, 61

Campylobacter, 37; in animal husbandry, 131
Candida, 37–38
Carbapenem-resistant Enterobacteriaceae (CRE), 35–36
Carbolic acid (phenol), 7–8

Chain, Ernest Boris, 9–10
Cleveland Clinic antibiotic
    guidelines, 100–101
Clinical balance sheet, 97
Clinical research stage, drug
    development process, 122–123
Clinic-based directly observed
    therapy (DOT), 113
Clostridium difficile (C. difficile),
    34–36
Colds, 61–63
Compound 606 (Salversan), 8–9
Conjugation (method of gene
    transfer), 16
Consequence tables, 96–97
Cystitis, 62

Decision tree, 97
Defined daily dose (DDD), 13
Destruction or inactivation (method
    of antimicrobial resistance),
    15–16
Developing countries: antibiotic use
    in animal husbandry, 136–138;
    antibiotic use in human
    medicine, 21–23
Development of new antibiotics,
    72–73; historical, 87–88;
    process, 88–89
Directly observed therapy (DOT), for
    tuberculosis, 112–114; Centers
    for Disease Control and
    Prevention (CDC)
    recommendations and
    procedures, 113; World Health
    Organization (WHO)
    recommendations, 113–114
Discovery and development phase,
    new drugs, 122
Disinfectants, 4
Doctors Without Borders (MSF),
    Ebola quarantine controversy
    and, 118–119
Domagk, Gerhard, 10

Drug development process, United
    States, 121–125; antibiotics
    and, 125–126
Drug quality and antimicrobial
    resistance, 23–14
Drug-resistant microbes, 14

Ebola, 71–72; air travel and,
    117–119; Centers for Disease
    Control and Prevention (CDC)
    guidelines for screening
    passengers, 118; state laws for
    screening passengers, 118–119;
    2014 outbreak, 117–119
Efflux (mechanism of antimicrobial
    resistance), 15
Ehrlich, Paul, 8–9
Emerging Infections program (EIP),
    Centers for Disease Control and
    Prevention (CDC), 74
Enterobacteriaceae, 38
Enterococci, 38; in animal husbandry,
    131–132
Escherichia coli (E. coli), 27, 33; in
    animal husbandry, 131
European regulation of antibiotics in
    animal husbandry, 128
Evolutionary pressure (selection
    pressure), 14–15

Factory farming and antibiotic use,
    129
Field-based directly observed therapy
    (DOT), 113
First-line drug, 14
Fleming, Alexander, 9
Florey, Sir Howard Walter, 9–10
Flu (influenza), 30; antiviral treatment
    for, 55; disease burden of, 54;
    vaccines, 54–55
Food and Drug Administration (FDA)
    (United States), drug
    development process and
    approval, 121–125

Generations of antibiotics (first-generation, second-generation, etc.), 5
Gene transfer, methods of, 16
Get Smart About Antibiotics (CDC program), 60
Gonococcal Isolate Surveillance Program (GISP), 74
Gonorrhea, 29; disease burden, 47; disease burden in the United States, 36–37; drug resistant, 48
Gram, Hans Christian, 6
Gram-positive and Gram-negative bacteria, 6–7
Gram staining, 6
Group B *Streptococcus* (GBS), 41–42
Growth promotion, antibiotic use in animal husbandry, 127–128; in Europe, 129–130; history, 129, 130
Guide to Good Prescribing, 98–99

Hand hygiene, 67
Healthcare-associated infection (HAI), 65–66; prevalence, 66–67
Herd immunity, 79–80
Hickox, Kaci, 118–119
HIV, 30, 51–52; drug resistance, 52–53; global burden of, 52
Horizontal gene transfer (lateral gene transfer), 16

Inappropriate use of antibiotics, 19–21
Individual and public approach to health and medical care, 111–112
Indoor residual spraying (IRS), 32–33
Infection control, 65–66; procedures, 67–68

Influenza (flu), 30; antiviral treatment for, 55; disease burden of, 54; vaccines, 54–55
Innovative Medicines Initiative, 89–90
Interventions to improve patient adherence, 108–110
In vitro and *in vivo* testing, 122

Klebsiella pneumoniae, 27, 33
Koch, Hermann Heinrich Robert, 11

Leprosy, quarantine and, 114–115
Lister, Joseph, 7–8

Malaria, 30–33; control of, 49; disease burden of, 49; drug resistant, 49–51
Meat, drug-resistant organisms in, 134–135
Medical decision making, 96–97
Medical Expenditure Panel Survey (MEPS), patterns of antibiotic use in the United States, 59–60
"The Medical Impact of the Use of Antibiotics in Food Animals" (WHO report, 1997), 130
Medication Adherence Clinical Reference (2011), 108–109
MedWatch, 124
Methicillin-resistant *Staphylococcus aureus* (MRSA): complications from, 33–34; prevalence, 40–41
Microbicides, 4
Microbistats, 4
Model List of Essential Medicines (WHO), 12
Multidrug-resistant microbes, 14
Mutation (mechanism of antimicrobial resistance), 15

Narrow-spectrum antimicrobials, 3–4

National Antimicrobial Resistance
Monitoring System
(NARMS), 74
National Healthcare Safety
Network, 60
National Pesticide Information Center
(Oregon State University), 4–5
National Quarantine Act (United
States), 117
National Tuberculosis Surveillance
Program (NTSS), 74–75
Neisseria gonorrhea (N. gonorrhea),
29; disease burden, 47; disease
burden in the United States,
36–37; drug resistant, 48
New Drug Application (NDA),
123–124

Obstacles to patient adherence,
106–108

Patent protection extension, 93
Patient adherence and nonadherence:
costs of nonadherence, 105;
defined, 103–104; difficulties in
measuring, 103–104; factors
related to, 105–106; rates of,
104–106
Penicillin, 9–10
Personal protective equipment (PPE),
67–68
Pharmacist education, 97–98
Pharyngitis (sore throat), 62
Phenol (carbolic acid), 7–8
Physician education, 97–99;
effectiveness of, 99–100;
passive and active strategies for,
99–100
Plague, quarantine and, 115–116
Pneumonia, 27–28, 33, 37–40
Postmarket safety monitoring, drug
approval process, 124–125
Preclinical research stage, drug
development process, 122

Prescribing practices, 57–59;
unnecessary use of antibiotics,
57–58; variations in antibiotics
use (Europe), 58–59; variations
in antibiotics use (United
States), 58–59
Prescription laws and access to
antibiotics, 20–22
Productivity in animal husbandry,
antibiotic use and, 135–136
Prontosil, 10
Prophylactic antibiotic use, animal
husbandry, 126
Pseudomonas aeruginosa, 38
Public health approach to health and
medical care, 111–112
Public health campaigns, 20–21

Quality of antibiotics, and drug
resistance, 23–14
Quarantine, 69–72; air travel and,
117–119; history of, 114–117;
internal, 117

Recommendations for antibiotic use,
United States, 84–87
Recommendations for antibiotic use,
World Health Organization
(WHO), 83–84
Research and development,
antibiotics: Europe, 89–90;
United States, 90–93
Review on Antimicrobial Resistance
(United Kingdom), 75–76
Rhinosinusitis, acute, 61–62

Salmonella, 28; in animal husbandry,
130–131; nontyphoidal, 38–39;
presence in meat for retail sale,
134–135; *Salmonella serotype
typhi*, 39
Salversan, 8–9
Sanitizers, 4
Second-line drugs, 14

Selection pressure (evolutionary
pressure), 14–15
Shigella, 28–29, 39
Smallpox, quarantine and, 116
Special Medical Use (SMU) pathway
for approval of new antibiotics,
91
Stakeholders in antibiotic use, 80–81
Staphylococcus aureus (S. aureus),
27–28; vancomycin-resistant,
40–41
Sterilizers, 4–5
Streptococcus, 40–42; Group B
(GBS), 41–42
*Streptococcus pneumoniae
(S. pneumoniae)*, 28
Streptomycin, 11–12
Sulfa drugs, 10–11
Surgery, antisepsis and, 7–8
Surveillance, recommendations for,
75–76
Surveillance and reporting programs,
73–75
Swann Committee (United Kingdom),
129
Syphilis, 8–9

Therapeutic antibiotic use, animal
husbandry, 127

Transduction (method of gene
transfer), 16
Transformation (method of gene
transfer), 16
Travel: and disease transmission,
69–70; Ebola and, 71;
multidrug-resistant tuberculosis
(MDR-TB) and, 71
Treatment adherence, 22–23
Treatment guidelines for antibiotic
use (CDC), 61–64
Tuberculosis, 11–12; disease burden,
United States, 44; disease
burden, worldwide, 44–45;
drug-resistant TB, 40, 44;
extensively drug-resistant
TB (XDR TB), 45–46;
multidrug-resistant TB
(MDR TB), 14, 29–30, 44;
quarantine of patients, 117;
treatment of, 44

Vaccination programs, 68–69
Vertical gene transfer, 16

Waksman, Selman Abraham, 11–12
Water pollution from antibiotic
plants, 81
World War II, penicillin and, 9–10

About the Author

Sarah E. Boslaugh, PhD, MPH, has worked for over 20 years as a researcher and statistician for various healthcare institutions, including Montefiore Medical Center in New York City and BJC HealthCare in St. Louis, Missouri. She is currently an adjunct professor of biostatistics at Saint Louis University, and has also taught at the Washington University School of Medicine (where she developed a two-semester statistics sequence for health professionals), the Program in Audiology and Communication Sciences at Washington University in St. Louis, and the department of psychological sciences at the University of Missouri-St. Louis. Dr. Boslaugh served as editor-in-chief for the *Encyclopedia of Epidemiology* (Sage, 2008) and the *Encyclopedia of Pharmacology and Society* (Sage, 2016), and has published numerous books, the most recent including *Statistics in a Nutshell* (2nd ed., O'Reilly, 2012) and *Health Care Systems Around the World: A Comparative Guide* (Sage, 2013).